Pregnancy Journal

A WEEK-BY-WEEK GUIDE TO A HAPPY, HEALTHY PREGNANCY

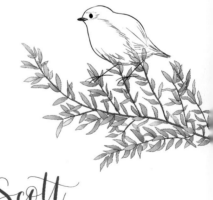

by Paula Spencer Scott

PETER PAUPER PRESS, INC.
Rye Brook, New York

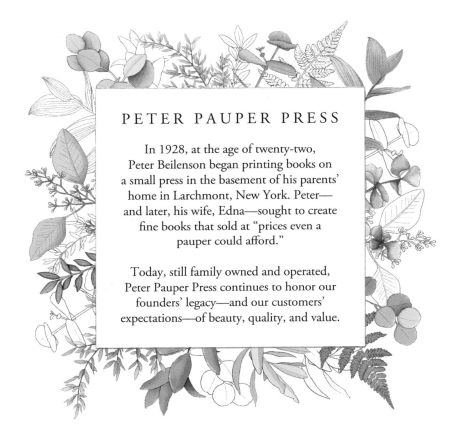

PETER PAUPER PRESS

In 1928, at the age of twenty-two,
Peter Beilenson began printing books on
a small press in the basement of his parents'
home in Larchmont, New York. Peter—
and later, his wife, Edna—sought to create
fine books that sold at "prices even a
pauper could afford."

Today, still family owned and operated,
Peter Pauper Press continues to honor our
founders' legacy—and our customers'
expectations—of beauty, quality, and value.

Designed by Heather Zschock

Copyright © 2024
Peter Pauper Press, Inc.
3 International Drive
Rye Brook, NY 10573 USA
ISBN 978-1-4413-4430-4
Printed in China

7 6 5 4 3 2 1

Visit us at www.peterpauper.com

Contents

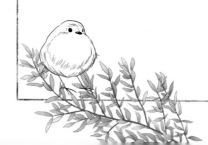
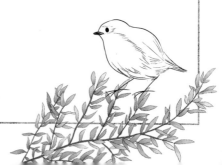

Introduction

• YOUR INCREDIBLE JOURNEY •

Welcome to an amazing, surprising, strange, thrilling, and topsy-turvy time of your life—nine months like no others.

Yes, that's a broad range of adjectives to link with pregnancy. But it's impossible to limit a description of the experience of having a baby to just a word or two.

And so this journal.

Because the journey from positive pregnancy test to full-fledged mom is filled with so much, it's helpful to have a special place to store your discoveries and your memories. Although no two pregnancies are alike, there's plenty of common ground in terms of topics you're apt to encounter. Ahead are great highs (like the first time you feel your baby move within you) as well as a few lows (like when nausea or a backache leaves you feeling a bit less glowy than the whole world seems to expect you to feel). And lots of wonders in between.

What you'll find here:

AN OUTLET. Use this journal as a place of refuge where you can write down the details of your incredible journey. Celebrate. Vent. Absorb. Mull. Marvel. Scribble lists or compose perfect sentences—whatever works for you. In addition to lots of writing space, we'll provide some "food for thought" prompts along the way.

A RECORD. To whom did you first break the news? When did you buy your first maternity top? What tests did you have, and when? Which names did you consider? Jot down key details for a permanent memento of your pregnancy story.

A KEEPSAKE. Use the inside back cover pocket to store such keepsakes as ultrasound photos, doctor's notes, and hospital wristbands.

A COMPANION. In these pages, you'll find helpful tips, insightful facts, fun ideas, and loads of empathy to smooth your progress from week to week.

A PREGNANCY GUIDE. Time-targeted, reliable information addresses your specific concerns along the way. We give an overview of the highlights that characterize each of the three trimesters of pregnancy, as well as dos and don'ts.

A WEEKLY SUPPORT SYSTEM. Then, for each week, we offer information about three different dimensions of pregnancy:

BABY UPDATE. How's he or she growing? What's happening in your womb this week?

BODY UPDATE. Advice and comfort tips on the physical side of being pregnant.

MIND UPDATE. Insights about possible mental, emotional, or other issues.

AN INSPIRATION. Quotations about pregnancy and motherhood sprinkled throughout these pages remind you that you're not alone—you're joining a league of mothers as old as (wo)mankind itself.

A word about how this journal counts the weeks.

The way that most doctors date a pregnancy, used here, is by **gestational age**, also called **menstrual age**. This means that the first official day of your pregnancy term is the first day of your last menstrual period (LMP). Conception usually occurs around two weeks after your LMP. So, when you are "13 weeks pregnant"—or in week 13 of this book—you have technically been pregnant for 11 weeks. Some doctors still use **fertilization age** (also called fetal age or ovulatory age, marking a pregnancy from the date you conceived), but since fertilization can be hard to pinpoint, dating by gestational age is considered more accurate.

Here's wishing you a healthy pregnancy
and happy journaling along the way.

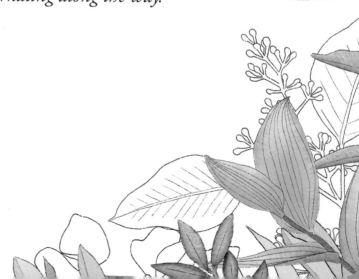

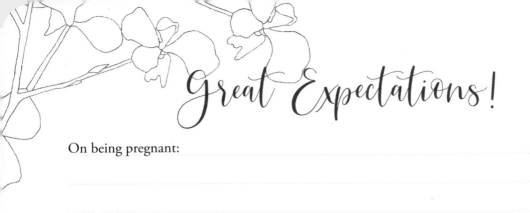

Great Expectations!

On being pregnant:

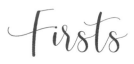

Firsts

First person I told the news to (who? when? how?)

....

....

....

When I first felt pregnant (and in what way)

....

....

First doctor visit

....

First heard the baby's heartbeat

....

When I first wore maternity clothes

....

First felt the baby move

....

Other firsts

....

....

....

A mother is always the beginning.
She is how things begin.

AMY TAN

WEIGHTS AND MEASUREMENTS

Pre-pregnancy weight:

WEEK	WEIGHT	WAIST
4		
6		
8		
10		
12		
14		
16		
18		
20		
22		
24		
26		
28		
30		
32		
34		
36		
37		
38		
39		
40		

TESTS AND RESULTS

TEST	DATE	RESULT

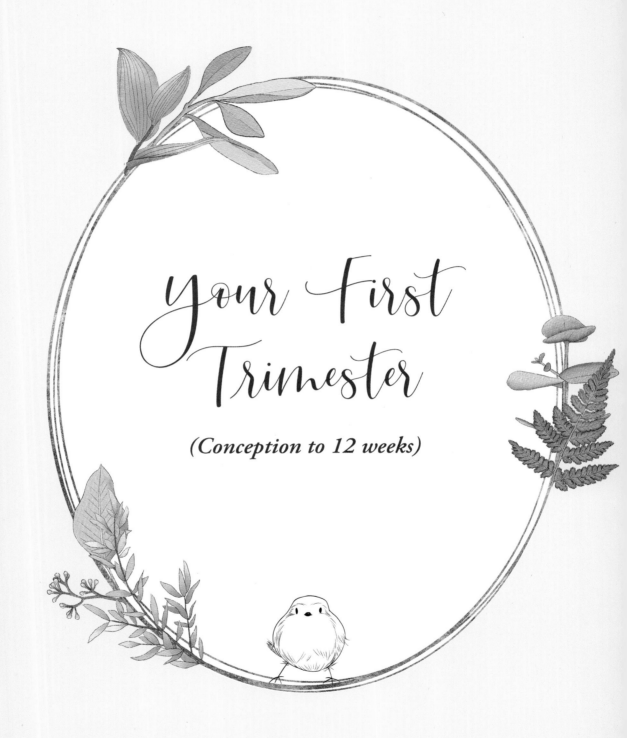

Your First
Trimester

(Conception to 12 weeks)

Off to a Great Start

All of pregnancy is a transition—but the first trimester feels especially so. These first weeks are all about getting used to the idea of being pregnant and doing what you can to safeguard the well-being of the new life you're carrying.

At first, it might not seem like much is happening; doubt, anxiety, or impatience sometimes race ahead of concrete physical signs. Then come the symptoms, catching up to your initial thoughts and, often, overtaking them. In a few brief weeks, you travel from the unreality of your big news to feeling that the pregnancy is unmistakably real.

One of the best predictors of a healthy baby is a healthy mother. Do what's in your power to give your baby a great head start. Now's a terrific time to shore up (or fine-tune) your health habits. What you eat or drink can affect your baby. So, how you spend your day—exercise, the kind of substances you handle, your stress level, and the amount of rest and relaxation you get—can influence the health of both of you.

Mostly, the first trimester is a time of getting things going: your health habits, your medical care, your support network, your baby plans, your idea of yourself as a pregnant woman. It's a lot to absorb. Luckily, pregnancy progresses one day at a time, giving you nine big months to make the mental and practical life adjustments you need.

First Trimester
DOS AND DON'TS

DO . . .

• **Make an appointment with an ob-gyn, midwife, or family doctor as soon as a home pregnancy test confirms the news.** The earlier you start receiving prenatal care, the better for you and your baby. You can expect to have a history taken, receive initial screenings and tests, get a prescription for prenatal vitamins, and (the best part) get an official due date!

• **Take your prescribed prenatal vitamins daily, if you can.** For some women, the added iron makes early nausea worse. Tip: Try taking the vitamin on a full stomach.

• **Start making shifts toward a healthier, well-balanced diet as soon as you know you are pregnant, if you haven't already.** Eat more plants, including nuts, beans, and legumes. Choose whole grains. Pick healthy fats (like olive oil, avocado, and fatty fish like wild salmon). Ideally, opt for grass-fed lean meats and dairy, which have a higher nutrition profile, and omega-3 fortified eggs. Avoid processed foods and fast food. But green-light all the fruits and veggies you like! The U.S. Food and Drug Administration advises pregnant women to avoid shark, swordfish, king mackerel, marlin, bigeye tuna, and tilefish because of mercury levels; limit albacore tuna to about 6 ounces per week. Get a nutritionist's input if you're vegan, vegetarian, lactose-intolerant, or have food allergies.

• **Target nutrients you especially need now.** They include:

Iron. Your body's need for it doubles in pregnancy, so many women become deficient. Found in dried fruits, grains, legumes, quinoa, and dark leafy vegetables.

Folate (folic acid). Helps prevent neural tube defects. Your prenatal vitamin contains it, but it's also found in bread, cereal, and pasta (which are fortified per U.S. government requirements), as well as legumes, soy, brewer's yeast, and dark leafy veggies.

Calcium. Builds fetal teeth and bones without depleting your reserves. Yogurt, milk, dark leafy greens, seeds, and salmon are sources.

Protein. Fuels fetal growth. Obtain via fish, lean meat, poultry, eggs, beans, nuts, lentils, wheat germ, and plain Greek yogurt.

• **Keep moving.** Most activities, other than scuba diving or sports with a high risk of falls, can be safely continued in the first trimester. The benefits to mood, baby, energy level, and overall well-being are tremendous! If you've never bothered much with workouts before but feel motivated now, good for you. Walking, swimming, and prenatal yoga are all perfect forms of exercise for pregnancy because you can continue them throughout your term.

• **Schedule X-rays after the first trimester,** if possible.

• **Report signs of bladder or urinary tract infection to your provider.** These include pain and burning when you pee, urgency, blood, or strong odor; you're at higher risk of UTIs especially in the first trimester, and the right treatment is important.

• **Enjoy couple time.** Make a point of doing things together and remember that this big change can seem more unreal to your mate, who, unlike you, doesn't "feel" any different.

• **Dream a little.** Sure, there's loads of medical advice and lots of planning right now. But it's also nice to take time to begin to imagine your future baby and your new family.

DON'T . . .

• **Don't smoke, vape, or spend time around people who are smoking.** Quitting in the first three months drops your risk of low birth weight to the same as a nonsmoker. Try a quit-smoking app for help, like quitSTART or QuitGuide.

• **Don't drink alcohol.** Although there's been lots of debate about how much is too much, most experts advise erring on the side of complete abstinence. Even "near beers" and nonalcoholic wines can contain some alcohol (unless they specify "alcohol-free").

• **Don't use other known damaging substances or services.** These include: marijuana, illegal drugs, douches, and tanning booths.

• **Don't overheat.** Skip hot tubs and hot yoga during pregnancy, as it's not a good idea to become overheated. Some doctors even nix electric blankets and long, hot soaks in the bath.

• **Don't handle or eat raw meat, raw seafood, and raw eggs,** to avoid bacteria and parasites. Also, skip sushi and sashimi; rare hamburgers or steaks; unpasteurized milk or juice; Caesar salad dressing or ice creams that contain raw eggs; unpasteurized cheese. Note: Almost all cheese sold in the U.S. is pasteurized, but if you're unsure, avoid soft cheeses made with raw milk like brie, feta, Camembert, queso blanco, and queso fresco.

• **Don't change cat litter.** Recruit someone else to do the job, since handling cat feces raises your risk of contracting the parasite that causes the infection toxoplasmosis. Also: wash your hands after handling a cat and keep cats off tables and countertops.

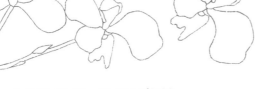

MORE DON'TS...

• **Don't be blithe about vitamins, supplements, and herbals.** Once you know you're pregnant, even before your first prenatal exam, call your doctor to discuss any prescriptions you now take. Certain acne medications, such as isotretinoin (formerly Accutane) and Retin-A (tretinoin), can harm a developing fetus. Many dietary supplements, herbs, and "natural" products are not government regulated and are often untested. That's why it's wise to run anything—including over-the-counter meds and botanicals advertised as safe for pregnancy—by your provider.

• **Don't "eat for two."** Your caloric needs barely rise in the first trimester—about the equivalent of an extra glass of milk—so don't feel like you need to increase your portions arbitrarily.

• **Don't go overboard on the baby gear (yet).** Give yourself this trimester to get a firm grounding on what's happening in your life first. You have weeks ahead to ogle and splurge!

• **Don't obsess too much over judgmental comments or scary warnings.** The biggies described above are important, but an occasional dietary slip-up or whiff of a passerby's cigar won't harm your baby. Really. Being relaxed is way more useful to your well-being than over-worry.

Conception

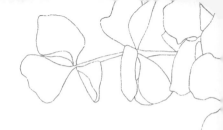

Meet Your New Zygote!

After sperm and egg unite, the egg closes its doors (in the form of its outer membrane) to other potential suitors. The precious baby you'll get to meet face-to-face in nine months has begun life as a zygote, a fertilized egg. It then multiplies into a tiny bunch of cells (about the size of the head of a pin) and is called a *blastocyst*. Within 3 or 4 days, this blastocyst burrows into the lining of your uterus so it can receive oxygen and nutrients and discard waste through your bloodstream. Its cells are also multiplying rapidly right now. By week 3, amniotic fluid (the "water" in "I think my water broke!"), which serves to cushion, warm, and protect your baby in the amniotic sac, has begun to surround it.

When's Your Due Date?

Pregnancy lasts about 38 weeks from conception to birth, or 40 weeks from the last menstrual period (LMP) to birth. To calculate your estimated due date, add 9 months and 7 days (a total of 280 days) to your LMP date.

Remember, though, that this due date is an estimate based on the average pregnancy. (A normal term can last between 37 to 42 weeks.) Most women (80 percent) give birth within 2 weeks of their due date—2 weeks before or 2 weeks after—but only about 4 to 5 percent deliver on their actual due date. As your pregnancy progresses, measurements of your uterus (fundal height), ultrasounds, and other physical observations will reinforce this due date and help your provider assess the progress of your pregnancy.

My first hints that I was pregnant

How I knew for sure

My reaction

My partner's reaction

Questions for my healthcare provider

Two weeks after we found out [I was pregnant], I played the Australian Open.
I told Alexis [Alexis Ohanian, her husband] it had to be a girl because
there I was, playing in 100-degree weather, and that baby never gave
me any trouble. Ride or die. Women are tough that way.

SERENA WILLIAMS

THE COUNTDOWN BEGINS

Week 4

Baby Update: SMALL MATTERS

By now, the blastocyst has divided into an embryo and a placenta. The embryo, which is your baby-to-be, is tinier than a grain of rice, with two distinct layers—the *epiblast* and *hypoblast*. As it grows, its cells will differentiate into specific jobs—the foundations for blood, nerves, and organs, for example.

The placenta is a very cool support system. This organ emerges to help produce hormones and to connect to the blood vessels in your uterine lining—all so it can, eventually, transfer oxygen and nutrients to your baby and discard released waste.

Body Update: FIRST SIGNS OF PREGNANCY

Many women notice changes in their breasts even before they miss a period. Your breasts may feel tender or larger, and the area around your nipples (areola) may look darker, larger, and/or bumpier. Breasts may tingle or feel more sensitive.

Sudden fatigue is another big clue. It can range from just-noticeable tiredness to flat-out exhaustion. You may begin feeling nauseated or bloated. Lots of women mistake these early symptoms for a case of the flu. Also common: A sudden aversion to smells or tastes that you never reacted to before (such as meat frying or chocolate). You may also feel the need to urinate more often.

Being "late" of course is the big bell-ringer. Some women will still see a little spotting, staining, or yellowish discharge around the time their period would be due.

False negatives are more common than false positives with home pregnancy tests. That's why, if you suspect you're pregnant, it's a good idea to wait a few days and re-test. Levels of the hormone hCG (*human chorionic gonadotropin*), produced by the pregnancy and detected by a pregnancy test, double every day in early pregnancy.

Mind Update: FIRST REACTIONS

Excited? Scared? Nervous? Ambivalent? Or are you still in a state of disbelief? These are perfectly natural first reactions to discovering that you are pregnant. There's no one "right" way to be. Give yourself a little time to absorb the news at the pace and way that feels right to you.

Don't be surprised if the way you feel isn't at all like what you expected. Maybe you tried so many months to get pregnant, and anticipated this big moment for so long, that its actuality is a bit of a letdown (especially if you're not feeling so hot). Maybe pregnancy caught you by surprise and you and your partner have mismatched reactions.

Many new mothers-to-be are so absorbed by their initial reactions to pregnancy—how they feel, what it means to their life, work, relationship, and plans—that they aren't even able to focus on the baby yet. Yup, that's normal too. Your becoming a mother is every bit as seismic as your having a baby. And while the two go hand-in-hand (obviously!), they're slightly different realities. Luckily you have ample time to get used to both.

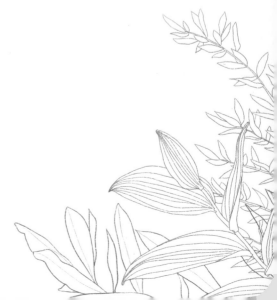

Am I Ready?

What I'm feeling right now

It's a really magical time, those first few weeks. It almost makes you wish you didn't have to tell anyone, ever. You could just watch your belly grow bigger, and no one would be allowed to ask you about it, and you would have your baby and a year later you would allow visitors to finally come and meet your little miracle.

AMY POEHLER

5 things I'm excited about

5 things I'm nervous about

Week 5

Baby Update

Your little embryo—that's what it's now called—is going through momentous changes. The embryo consists of three layers: *ectoderm*, *endoderm*, and *mesoderm*. As befits their sci-fi names, each has a futuristic job to do. The ectoderm will develop into the brain and nervous system, skin, hair, nails, tooth enamel, and mammary and sweat glands. The endoderm will develop into the lungs, gastrointestinal tract, pancreas, thyroid, and liver. And the mesoderm will become the heart and circulatory system, skeleton, blood system, urogenital system, and the muscles and connective tissues.

Already this week, your baby's heart begins to beat regularly; arm and leg buds appear; and the eyes, ears, and skeleton begin to form. The placenta and umbilical cord begin to function around this time, too.

Body Update: THE ART OF LISTENING TO YOUR BODY

When you're tired, do you nap, or at least put your feet up? When your stomach is full, do you stop eating? These are common examples of listening to your body. That's an important skill during pregnancy, because your trusty, hardworking body has a lot to tell you. The changes that every system within you will experience in the coming months are tremendous. If you try to plow on ahead as if there's "nothing different," you're denying reality—actual physical need.

Slow down a little bit and hear what your body wants to say. Its aches and pains might be telling you to ease up on certain activities, to stretch or have a massage, or to sleep in a different position. If certain smells or tastes are suddenly objectionable, avoid them. (It's no coincidence that many women report disliking the smell of cigarettes or the taste of alcohol in pregnancy, both things that are known to negatively affect a growing fetus.)

Your body will tell you what it likes, too! You might find yourself calmed and soothed by sitting quietly and rubbing your belly, for example. A morning walk might pep you up and quell nausea all day long. The advice of doctors and pregnancy guidebooks boils down to suggestions that have been shown to work for most women. But only you have your body, and only you can hear what it wants most from you.

Mind Update: SPREADING THE NEWS, MAYBE

Whom will you tell that you're pregnant, and when? It's very personal! Some parents-to-be are inclined to share their happy news with the world (or, at least, everyone they know) as soon as a pregnancy test confirms it. Others prefer to keep mum for a while. They may simply want to keep this very special secret between themselves for a few precious weeks or prefer to wait until the greatest danger of miscarriage is past, usually between 9 and 12 weeks.

Some newly expectant mothers compromise. They confide in a close friend, sister, or their own mother, to have someone with whom they can talk or compare notes (besides their partner). Then they wait a bit longer to tell other friends and family members, colleagues, and casual acquaintances.

How will you make the big announcement? In a series of elated phone calls? At a big "surprise" party? A fun Instagram bombshell? Different audiences might warrant different approaches. At work, you might want to have a confidential talk with your human resources representative first, to discuss options about maternity leave and benefits, so that you can better formulate a plan to present to your supervisor when you tell her.

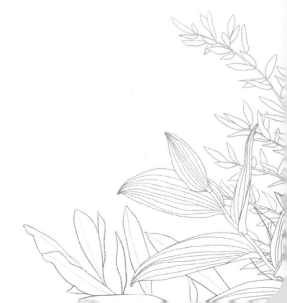

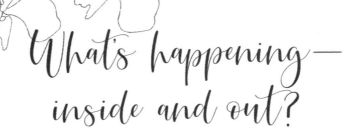

What's happening— inside and out?

Who knows, so far

Reactions

Announcement ideas

It is the most powerful creation for you to be able to have life growing inside of you.
There is no bigger gift, nothing more empowering.

BEYONCÉ

Week 6

Baby Update

This week your speck of a baby is barely 1/4 inch (0.6 cm) long—picture a dried pea in the shape of a curled tadpole. (The measurement of your baby's length is now calculated from the crown of the head to the buttocks because the legs are curled close to the chest.) Arms and legs are becoming longer and they now grow hand and feet buds, with tiny, webbed fingers and toes. Your baby's jaw, tongue, nose, and lungs also begin to form. Muscle fibers are starting to grow, and your baby's intestines and brain continue to develop.

It's possible to hear your baby's heartbeat (going much faster than your own—about 100 to 130 beats per minute) with a vaginal ultrasound. It's working hard to circulate blood to support all this rapid growth.

Body Update: EASING EARLY DISCOMFORTS

Hollywood's favorite pregnancy ailments are morning sickness (which is common) and fainting (which is rare), but you're probably feeling other strange stuff, too. Luckily, there are things you can do to feel better.

If you suffer from gas, bloating, and heartburn: Avoid fried and fatty foods, or those that produce gas, like beans, cruciferous veggies, and dairy. Eat slowly. A leisurely walk after a meal—even if it's just around your house—can also help.

If your breasts feel swollen and sore: Try a new bra that fits better and gives you more support. You may need several bra updates during your pregnancy, so err on the side of roominess when you choose one. Avoid underwires, which can pinch or even compress mammary glands. Sports bras can be great. Some women are helped by wearing a bra to sleep.

If you're getting headaches: Try nonmedical treatments first, such as fresh air, rest, or a relaxation technique. Acetaminophen used to be considered safe in pregnancy but recent studies have doctors unsure; it's best to avoid it—as well as aspirin, ibuprofen, and other medications—without medical approval. If headaches are persistent or severe, tell your doctor.

If increased vaginal discharge bothers you: Try wearing a panty liner and changing it often. Cotton underwear tends to be more comfortable than synthetic.

If you're congested: This is an unexpected but common side effect of pregnancy. Try using a humidifier and elevating your head when you sleep. Drink lots of fluids. Don't take antihistamines or other cold medications without your doctor's okay.

Mind Update: EXPECTING CHANGE

"Your life will never be the same." Heard that yet? Don't let it unnerve you. As ominous as the sentiment might sound, it's based in truth—here's why it really will be okay.

It's true a baby will likely keep you from some enjoyable activities you're used to, especially in the first few months. You may be so distracted by your new priorities, however, that you don't miss the activities as much as you might have expected. Once you "pay your dues" taking care of a newborn, you can begin to bring some of those activities back. Plus, you get to spend time playing, cuddling, and finding joy in unexpected ways.

Sleep deprivation is not a myth. Your newborn will need you constantly, at all hours of the day and night, for food, soothing, diaper changes, and even help getting to sleep. Take comfort knowing that the more you respond to your baby's needs, the more he learns to trust and love you. What seems thankless, early on, is setting the stage for future emotions and learning. Once your baby starts smiling (around six weeks), it all seems so much easier!

Even though much of your day will be dedicated to taking care of your baby, there are ways to make time for yourself and other relationships. You and your partner will get to see and admire whole new sides of each other, too. So yes, big changes are ahead, but, on balance, the gains outnumber the losses.

DID YOU KNOW that you may be referred to as an "elderly primigravida" if you are only in your 30s? It simply means you are an "older" (in obstetrical terms) first-time mother. Maternal age is just one factor that doctors use to determine how often you'll need ultrasounds or other checkups.

My support squad

Mom role models

Likes and dislikes

*Giving birth and being born brings us into the essence of creation,
where the human spirit is courageous and bold and the body,
a miracle of wisdom.*

HARRIETTE HARTIGAN

Week 7

Baby Update

Your embryo is still tiny but—ta da!—reaches the size of a small berry, about half an inch (1.3 cm). Her head is bigger than her body, with dark spots where the eyes will form. She can already move in the amniotic sac. Fingers and toes are separating, and elbows are now visible. Vital organs are developing, as well as fine details: teeth, eyelids, nipples, and hair follicles. The liver is now producing red blood cells, and blood vessels in the umbilical cord represent your baby's lifeline—carrying oxygen and nutrients between the two of you.

Body Update: *NAUSEA HELPERS*

Morning sickness peaks from weeks 7 to 12, generally—but its timing and severity vary considerably from woman to woman. Morning sickness is the worst-named condition of pregnancy. You can feel sick to your stomach any time of the day, or even all day. Symptoms do tend to be worst first thing in the morning for many women.

Nobody knows exactly what causes nausea and vomiting, or why its intensity can be so different from one woman to another. (Up to 90 percent of moms-to-be experience it.) Hormonal changes are almost certainly a trigger. Discomfort eases, in all but a small percentage of cases, by the end of the first trimester. Even better news: Your misery doesn't bother your baby a bit, and nausea has been found to signal a lower risk of miscarriage. (It's also true that you can have NO sickness and your baby will be fine.)

Some tactics that can help in the meantime:

• **Eat strategically.** Don't avoid food completely when nausea strikes, because this can make you feel worse. Try small, light meals, and keep a stash of plain, dry snacks such as crackers, rice cakes, or cereal on hand for nibbling. If you eat a little before you feel hungry, you may be able to stave off an attack. Avoid heavily sauced foods, junk food, or greasy items as they're slow to digest.

• **Stay vertical.** Lying down immediately or soon after eating can make you queasy. Snack when you wake up in the morning, before getting out of bed. If you can, stay in bed sitting upright for about 15 minutes before getting up. Snack again before you go to bed.

• **Drink lots of water and other fluids.** Dehydration can exacerbate nausea.

• **Give your nose a break.** Avoid stuffy rooms by keeping windows open. Because strong smells can trigger nausea, remove highly scented soaps, perfumes, and foods from your home.

• **Try ginger.** So-called "pregnancy teas" and botanical tonics are unregulated and untested, and can cause serious side effects, even miscarriage. Exception: A cup or two of ordinary ginger tea (or you can grate a little fresh ginger in hot water). Ginger, like two other herbs good for tea, peppermint and spearmint, has been shown to calm queasiness.

• **Try acupressure bands.** Sold over-the-counter, these wristbands have a plastic disc that rests on your pressure point. They're advertised for motion sickness and seasickness, but are a low-tech remedy for pregnancy sickness as well.

• **Consult with your doctor if:** You vomit more than twice a day, can't keep anything down at all, or seem to be dropping weight quickly. A small percentage of women suffer especially severe morning sickness (called *hyperemesis gravidarum*, or *HG*), which warrants close supervision to avoid dehydration and other problems.

Mind Update: REMEMBER WHEN . . . ?

It's hard to believe, but nine months from now your pregnancy will probably become a blur. In addition to your journal, consider preserving some of your memories of this special time. Your family will love looking back. Some ideas:

• **Write a letter to your baby.** Tell your baby how you feel about meeting and getting to know them and what you look forward to doing with them. Share your hopes and dreams for them. Ask your partner to write something, too. Reading each other's letters has the added benefit of giving one another insights into your feelings now.

• **Track your changing shape.** Choose one day of each month (the first, the last) and have someone photograph you or take a selfie. (Profiles are especially dramatic.)

• **Start a memory box.** Use any cute container or the inside back cover pocket of this book to keep mementos: ultrasound printouts, doctors' notes, shower invitations, doodled lists of all those baby names, etc.

Dear Baby,

Love,

When I listen to my body, it says

When I listen to my heart, it says

To be pregnant is to be vitally alive, thoroughly woman, and distressingly inhabited. Soul and spirit are stretched—along with body—making pregnancy a time of transition, growth, and profound beginnings.

ANNE CHRISTIAN BUCHANAN

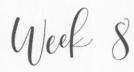

Week 8

Baby Update

Not yet an inch (2.5 cm) long, your baby is taking on a more familiar human shape. The body straightens out a bit and the head becomes more erect. The embryonic "tail" is receding (it will eventually be the tailbone). The limbs, fingers, and toes are getting longer and—aw—the hands reach for each other over the heart. Facial features are becoming more distinct, too, and nerve cells in your future Brainiac's brain are feverishly wiring up.

Body Update: VITAMINS AND SUPPLEMENTS

Your baby depends on you for nutrients, vitamins, and minerals vital to growth and development. For this reason, your doctor has probably recommended a special prenatal vitamin. Reinforce the daily habit by taking it at the same time each day, such as after breakfast. That timing has the added advantage of lessening the likelihood of nausea, since you'll have something in your stomach. Taking your vitamin with orange juice helps your body better absorb the iron in it. Another way to remember: Keep the bottle next to your toothbrush or hairbrush where you'll see it, linking the two habits.

Vitamins and minerals are most readily absorbed in their natural form, though, so you want to keep swallowing all those plant-based nutrients and fish, too. Prenatal supplements don't include the full recommended allowance of certain nutrients, such as protein and calcium.

You do need to be careful with vitamins, though. Don't take two doses in one day to "catch up" if you miss a day. Certain vitamins, such as vitamin A, can be dangerous in amounts over the recommended daily allowance (more than 10,000 IU of vitamin A is toxic). There are cases where your doctor might suggest a supplement, such as added iron in the event of anemia, or extra calcium. Follow medical advice in this area rather than self-treating.

Mind Update: HOW TO GET THE MOST OUT OF CHECK-UPS

How do you like your care provider so far? You'll get better, more personalized care if you like and respect one another. If you're not on the same page philosophically, or just don't mesh, better to make a change at this point in your pregnancy.

Some ways to make your appointments better:

• **Keep a list of questions and concerns in a handy place, such as in your phone or in this journal.** Then you won't forget them. Bring the list to your appointment and don't let yourself get rushed out before you ask away. It's proactive, not obsessive!

• **Ask questions, no matter how dumb or embarrassing they may seem.** Your care provider has heard everything before, but you haven't, and that's what matters.

• **Clarify anything you don't completely understand.** Try repeating what your provider tells you in your own words to make sure you've got it right.

• **Double-check with your provider what you read or hear about pregnancy if you want to be sure about something.** Don't just take Google's or your mother's word for it.

• **Prod your doctor or midwife further if something she's said doesn't seem right to you.** Remember you're a team, and your own instincts are useful guides.

• **Take notes during your appointments.** If your partner comes, that's two sets of ears.

• **Try not to act defensive.** The medical team isn't asking about your habits or lifestyle to be nosy, and isn't putting you on the scale to be judgmental. It's all useful info.

• **Accept handouts.** Pick up brochures on pregnancy. Written information that you can read over at your leisure may clarify points made during appointments.

• **Be honest, open, and specific when you describe how you feel.** Here is one place where you should drop the "happy mask" and be candid. Speak up if you're feeling scared, sad, or anxious; battling an eating disorder; having relationship trouble; concerned about any condition you have; or feeling depressed or anxious (or have a history of these conditions).

DID YOU KNOW that your clothes might feel tight in the waist weeks before you "show"?

My emotional weather report

What I'm eating now

How I'm exercising now

My latest questions

Being a mother redefines us, reinvents us, destroys and rebuilds us. Being a mother brings us face-to-face with ourselves as children, with our mothers as human beings, with our darkest fears of who we really are. Being a mother requires us to get it together or risk messing up another person forever.

SHONDA RHIMES

Week 9

Baby Update

Your baby is now about 1 to 1-1/4 inches (2.5 to 3.2 cm) long and will begin to gain weight at a quicker pace. The eyes are now covered by full eyelids (which won't open until around 28 weeks), and the pupils and optic nerve are developing. Other facial features—nose, lips, and mouth—are also becoming more defined.

Your baby can now move arms, legs, hands, and feet better since all the joints work and the muscles can contract. Most of the time, though, she prefers to stay curled up.

Body Update: *RELAXING MOVES*

Pregnant women tend to receive a lot of information and advice, but surprisingly little about relaxation. Relaxing isn't just something that helps you mentally. It has physical benefits, too. When you relax, your body can rest and revive itself. Breathing slows, muscles lose their tension, stress endorphins stop racing through your system, your heart rate slows—a set of remarkable physical changes occurs, known as the relaxation response. With all that your body has going on right now, giving it a chance to take a break is both restorative and healing.

Experiment to see what works for you:

• **Yoga.** Look for a non-heated class or videos tailored to pregnant women.

• **Breathing exercises.** Deep, slow breathing for just a few minutes can trigger the relaxation response.

• **Mindfulness or meditation.** If you're new to a practice or under a lot of stress, look for a course in mindfulness-based stress reduction or download a mindfulness or guided meditation app.

• **Get outside.** Try walking in the park or have a picnic in fresh air.

• **Massage.** Avoid deep work and, ideally, find someone experienced with treating pregnant women.

• **Progressive muscle relaxation.** Starting at your head and, working down, tense up and then release each major muscle group.

• **Journaling.** Try just sitting quietly and writing about something positive, like your wishes for your unborn child.

Mind Update: ALL ABOARD THE EMOTIONAL ROLLER COASTER

One minute you're so excited you don't know how you can wait until your delivery day. The next, you're in tears. Emotional ups and downs are vivid during the first trimester. Blame hormones, in part. Their levels change dramatically as your baby forms and your body prepares for childbirth. Add a good bit of stress as all the pieces of your life slowly change. All this and excitement, too! It's all so dramatic—and yet so abstract, too.

What helps: Recognizing that your conflicting feelings are typical. So what if everyone is expecting you to be glowing and cheerful 24/7 (while, for at least some of those hours, you're neither)? Having friends to confide in can make a huge difference. Your partner may be such a person, but also sometimes may be part of the problem on a given day. Other women who have been through pregnancy before can provide a great outlet. If you're still keeping your condition a secret, join an online community of pregnant women.

DID YOU KNOW that it's safe to get a flu shot in pregnancy? In fact, government health agencies recommend it for all pregnant women prior to flu season, each November to March. (Note: If you are allergic to eggs, check with your doctor first.) COVID-19 vaccines and yearly boosters are also safe to receive (and recommended!) during pregnancy.

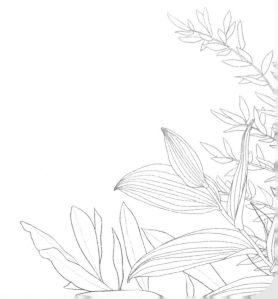

What calms me and brings me back to center

I am in love with a human
I haven't met yet.

AUTHOR UNKNOWN

Week 10

Baby Update

This week, your baby's body is about 1-1/2 inches (3.8 cm) long, with the head taking up about half of that. Weight: around 1/4 ounce (7 g). Your baby's head's size and bulging shape reflect how tremendously the brain is growing and maturing. Most vital organs have begun to function. Spinal nerves are branching out from the spinal cord.

Although you can't feel it yet, your baby is very active despite the still-minuscule size. More big news: By the end of the week, your baby's officially known as a fetus.

Body Update: CRAVINGS

Chocolate? Peppermint ice cream? Pickled okra? It's not just folklore. Many mothers-to-be find that they hunger for particular foods early in their pregnancy. Some evolutionary biologists believe that cravings, as well as aversions, are the way your pregnant body tells you which foods are desirable or not. (In caveman days, for example, meat with a strong odor might have signaled rot—not good for a baby on board.) Nobody knows for sure, but preferences are also affected by hormones and altered senses of taste and smell.

Some cravings may in fact lead you toward food choices rich in nutrients, such as fresh fruits or milk. Other cravings may lead you toward sweet, salty, or carb-filled meals and snacks. Whatever the craving, go slow, and focus on which foods leave you feeling best, both physically and mentally. If certain snacks leave you feeling sick or sluggish, don't be afraid to experiment with alternatives that also satisfy—a cup of hot chocolate instead of a candy bar—or additions that make snacks more satiating—nut butters or fresh fruit with your craving of choice.

Remember—your body is doing incredible work. Don't diminish it by denying yourself. You deserve food that satisfies your body and spirit.

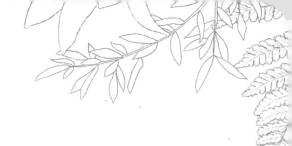

Mind Update: *TEST ANXIETY*

Prenatal testing is a double-edged sword: Each test is an opportunity to offer reassurance that all's well, and another thing to worry about. It's certainly normal to feel anxious about your baby's well-being. And waiting for results, as well as thinking about next steps in the event of a potential problem, can be nerve-wracking.

Meet your anxiety halfway by being informed. Get clear about why a test is being offered to you, how it's done, and how and when the results will be conveyed. Be aware of the difference between a screening test (such as the First Trimester Screen), which looks for clues to the possibility of a problem, and a diagnostic test (such as amniocentesis or chorionic villus sampling), which can diagnose one.

Remind yourself that most health problems are caused by genetics or quirks of fate or unknown causes—not something that the mother did or did not do. Birth defects are often correctable.

If you're anxious about a particular test, talk it through with your care provider. She can help you weigh the risks and benefits through the lens of your situation. Be aware that it's your right to refuse a test.

DID YOU KNOW that chocolate is the most craved food in the U.S.? Top craves vary widely by culture.

Likes and dislikes

Cravings

Sensitivities

Now my belly is as noble as my heart.

GABRIELA MISTRAL

Week 11

Baby Update

Now 2 inches (5.1 cm) long, your baby weighs around 1/3 of an ounce (9.4 g). Under paper-thin and transparent skin, the skeleton is starting to harden as bone replaces cartilage. Little tooth buds are forming under the gums (though the first tooth won't appear until 4 to 7 months post-birth). Your baby's got skills: thumb-sucking, kicking, swallowing amniotic fluid, stretching, and body surfing. He might also experience—though they'll be imperceptible to you—bouts of hiccups, which make his entire body bounce.

Body Update: *FEW GROUNDS FOR SHAME ON CAFFEINE*

If you're a java junkie, you've probably already discovered that a cup or two of joe per day (about 200 mg caffeine) is generally considered well within safe limits. Caffeine can slightly raise your blood pressure, add to heartburn, keep you awake, and possibly dehydrate you. Some studies have linked excessive caffeine, about three or more cups of coffee a day, to an increased risk of miscarriage. So, all-day Starbucks is out, but most docs now okay a wake-up cup.

Be mindful of overall caffeine intake in a day. The amount of caffeine in black tea steeped for a minute or less, or in chocolate, isn't significant, unless you consume huge quantities. (It's also in some sodas, but you don't want to be drinking those anyway.)

Ideally, switch to decaf coffee or decaf or herbal tea. Wean yourself from a serious caffeine habit with half-caffeinated brews, gradually tapering off the amount that's caffeinated, to avoid withdrawal symptoms such as headaches and fatigue.

If you miss the energy boost you get from caffeine, try exercising more or having a protein-rich snack instead. If you're used to sipping all day long, start carrying a sports bottle with water as a replacement.

Mind Update: COPING WITH WELL-INTENTIONED "ADVICE"

Some words of wisdom tilt more to the wacky than the wise. Listen and laugh, and when in doubt, ask your provider.

Consider three old wives' tales:

• You can tell the sex of your baby by looking for "signs."

False: Although it might be fun to guess boy or girl by examining your freckles or the position of your "bump," there's no accuracy to these methods—despite what Great-Aunt Martha says.

• Stress can hurt your baby.

Semi-true: The moderate levels of stress that come with most everyday challenges—deadlines, traffic, fights with your loved ones—isn't what researchers worry about. Most mothers-to-be don't live in placid plastic bubbles, after all. There is, however, some evidence linking extreme or prolonged stress to premature birth or low birth weight, which is why it's worth confiding to a doctor or midwife about a super-stressful situation in your life, whether work or personal.

• You will injure your baby if you have sex.

Pretty Much False: Your baby is well protected by the amniotic sac and uterus, and therefore unaffected by intercourse. Exception: Your doctor may advise against sex in certain high-risk pregnancy situations, mostly just as a precaution.

DID YOU KNOW that partners get weepy, gain weight, and crave ice cream too? "Couvade syndrome" (a.k.a. sympathetic pregnancy) spikes now and can last to Delivery Day.

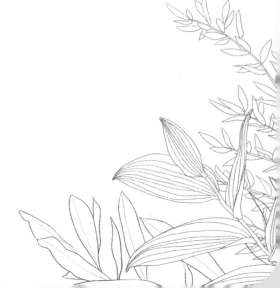

Weird advice I've been given

Good advice I want to remember

My favorite sources of pregnancy info so far

Let us make pregnancy an occasion when we appreciate our female bodies.

MERETE LEONHARDT-LUPA

Week 12

The first trimester ends. Great news: the likelihood of a miscarriage drops sharply.

Baby Update

Pea pod indeed! That's about how long your baby is—2-1/2 inches (6.4 cm)—with a face that's starting to organize itself into that of a newborn. The intestines, which grew so fast that they spilled into the umbilical cord, now retreat into the abdominal cavity. Also around this time, her kidneys start excreting urine. As the nervous system continues to develop, your baby can blink, kick, and wriggle.

Body Update: *GETTING A GOOD NIGHT'S SLEEP*

Even if you haven't gained much weight yet, you may find it difficult to sleep comfortably. Tactics that help:

• **Lie on your left side.** Side sleeping is comfier, and the left side is most beneficial for your baby because it best supports the flow of blood and nutrients to the placenta. Bend your knees, too.

• **Tuck a pillow between your knees and anywhere else that helps you feel supported and comfortable, such as under your belly or behind your back.** Some mothers-to-be swear by a long body pillow.

• **Around this point in your pregnancy, it's important to avoid sleeping on your back.** This position exerts pressure on the inferior vena cava (a major artery), which impedes circulation, as well as on your intestines and on your back. You should also avoid stretching or exercising in this position until after you deliver.

• **Fine-tune your sleep setup as your pregnancy progresses.** You may want to add or rearrange support pillows as you get bigger, for example. You may also feel warmer, and therefore need fewer covers or bedclothes, or a lower thermostat setting.

Mind Update: *PICKING A NAME*

Sometimes it takes a full 40 weeks for a couple to agree!

Among the considerations: Original or traditional? Gender specific or gender neutral? Do you want to honor someone or pick a name that reflects something meaningful to you? Will you call the child by the formal version of the name, or a nickname? Are there alternative spellings to consider? What about a middle name? Or two? And how will you handle the last name?

Among the places to look for ideas: Name-finder tools and name generators; your family tree; historical or current public figures; favorite books or shows; fairy tales; nature guides; the Bible; an atlas; a "love map" of your favorite places; old phone books at the library; the Social Security Administration site for lists of names by decade or state; groupthink (if you dare!).

Play the name game: Every week, you each make a separate list of 3 to 5 favorites. On Sunday nights, compare them. Any double wins worth considering?

Then you'll have to decide whether you'll share your picks with the world before your baby is born. Some parents like to do this because they prefer to address their unborn child by his or her actual name throughout pregnancy, to feel more closely bonded. Others prefer to wait until the name is attached to their living breathing newborn. That way friends and relatives are less likely to criticize the name.

TOP BABY NAME CONTENDERS

	My favorites	My partner's favorites
Boy:		
Girl:		

Why I like these

_____

_____

DID YOU KNOW that one in five moms later regret their baby's name? For 11 percent of "name remorse" moms, the name proved too hard to spell or pronounce.

Baby registry planner: early wish list

Favorite playlist right now

Favorite pregnancy snack now

First trimester wrap-up: What I'm thinking about right now

There is such a special sweetness in being able to participate in creation.

PAMELA S. NADAVA

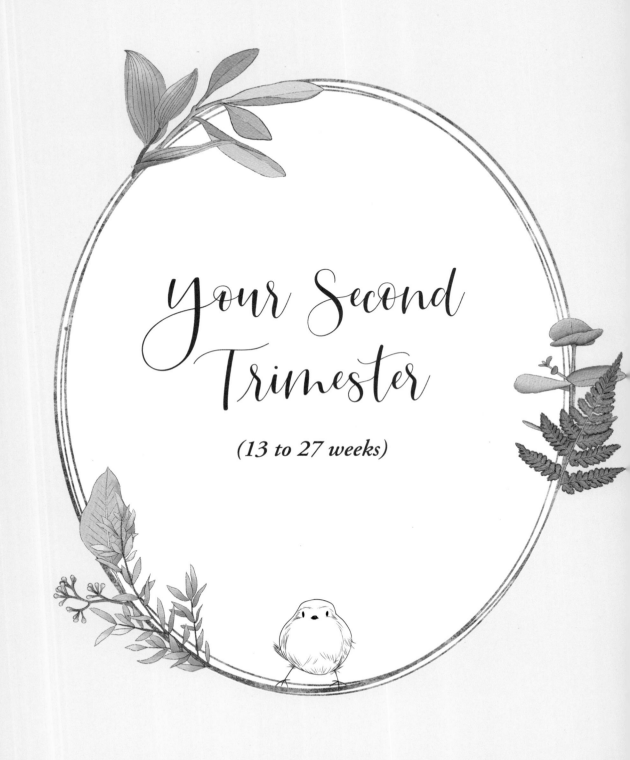

Your Second Trimester

(13 to 27 weeks)

The Middle of Everything

For most women, the middle of pregnancy is relatively calm. Initial adjustments, weird aversions, and tender breasts recede, while an unwieldy body and labor pains are still far off. Energy tends to pick up; nausea subsides. Your bump becomes noticeable and fun to dress. And many women enjoy having curves, lusher hair, and brighter skin.

Not that it's all a party. Some women continue to suffer pregnancy sickness and other random complaints or develop complications that bear watching. (Sorry.) It's also perfectly normal to feel ambivalent or apprehensive about what's happening. That's the thing about being pregnant—you have to be receptive to whatever the reality of it turns out to be for you.

Your thoughts begin to shift from what's-happening-in-my-body to who's-that-in-my-body as you start to feel the baby move. Talking to your baby, referring to him or her by name (or a made-up, in-utero pet name), or patting your belly are all the beginnings of bonding.

Becoming more aware of your baby can make smart health choices easier. Talk about a powerful motivation!

Second Trimester

DOS AND DON'TS

DO . . .

• **Enjoy the bloom and bursts of energy, as they come.** Admire your changing shape in the mirror and keep taking weekly side-selfies.

• **Continue taking prenatal vitamins as recommended.** The iron, folic acid, calcium, and other nutrients are important all through pregnancy.

• **Focus on protein.** Your body needs it to help fuel your baby's development. Beyond the usual meat sources, consider eggs, tofu and other soy products, Greek yogurt, Icelandic yogurt (skyr), wheat germ, nuts, nut butters, cheese, fish, and the countless variety of beans.

• **Use common sense when exercising.** Stretch beforehand. Quit when you become overexerted and don't allow yourself to become overheated. Drink water before and after your workout. If you're too sick or tired to exercise, don't force it; give yourself an occasional break.

• **Take advantage of the "sexy surge" if it happens to you.** Surging hormones and more blood flow to the pelvis often make women feel especially frisky in the middle months. Consider it one of the fringe benefits of pregnancy.

• **Get key to-do list items out of the way.** Get your teeth cleaned, have an eye exam, have your car inspected, write or update your will with the baby in mind.

• **Wear a seat belt in the car every time.** Position the lap strap just below your belly (not across it) and the diagonal strap between your breasts. If the shoulder strap is uncomfortable, raise or lower your seat—please don't just move the strap under your arm.

• **Enjoy 1-on-1 outings with your partner.** Go to a movie, eat out, plan a babymoon.

DON'T . . .

• **Don't eat for two.** Eat for you. Listen to your body, and focus on eating foods that give you energy and keep you satisfied.

• **Don't believe everything you hear.** There's nothing like a visibly pregnant woman to invite advice, comments, and strange-but-supposedly-true tales of how to determine an unborn baby's gender, health, or personality. Take everything you're told by well-intentioned (but not necessarily medically trained) observers with two grains of salt.

• **Don't expect to feel like anybody else.** Comparing notes with other pregnant women can be helpful, but only to a point. The range of symptoms and issues is so broad and individualized that it's impossible to tell you how you should be feeling at any given time.

• **Don't leave your care provider out of the loop.** If you become interested in an alternative therapy, whether it's a botanical product, hypnosis, acupuncture, sound therapy, or something else, consult your doctor or midwife. These treatments can work with, or against, your conventional medical treatment. Ideally, those treating you should be on the same page. Be aware that some alternative therapies are unstudied in pregnancy.

• **Don't overdo it.** Now's a season for lightening your overall load, not adding to it. Take breaks more often than you used to, and make sure you get at least 7 to 8 hours' sleep at night. If you want to throw a gender-reveal party, go for it—but if the idea of arranging a color-coordinated cake and balloons makes you want to nap . . . skip it and nap.

• **Don't miss obstetric visits if you feel fine.** It's important for your health and your baby's to be monitored at the regular intervals recommended by your doctor or midwife.

My second-trimester to-do list

Questions for my health provider

One of the most exciting things about being pregnant is that I just am accepting the complete unknown; it's a complete mystery and miracle.

N ATALIE P ORTMAN

Week 13

Good news! Expect nausea to suddenly lift as hCG levels stabilize.

Baby Update

Measuring about 3 inches (7.6 cm) and weighing around 1 ounce (23.4 g), your baby looks a bit like a miniature—very miniature—newborn. The little body is fully formed, though his head is still disproportionately large. His kidneys and urinary tract are fully functioning this week: He can swallow and expel amniotic fluid. Most of the critical development of the organs and body systems is complete. One tiny detail is also complete—your baby even has unique fingerprints. Over the next six months, the focus is on growing larger and stronger for survival outside of you.

Body Update: DENTAL CARE

It's a myth that you should avoid the dentist during pregnancy. To the contrary, keeping your mouth clean and healthy is important for both you and your baby. A surprising number of infections begin orally. Some women prefer to schedule a checkup during the second trimester once morning sickness abates.

Just a few precautions: Avoid X-rays if possible. If you need to have them done, wear a lead shield for protection. Also, if you need dental work beyond a regular cleaning, discuss the safety of the procedure and the anesthesia it requires with your doctor beforehand; some procedures can be easily postponed until after delivery.

Focus on daily dental care at home because you're more prone to gum infections when pregnant, which can affect your baby. Brush your teeth (and gums) with a soft-bristle brush and floss regularly. Gums tend to be more sensitive and bleed more easily in pregnancy, but don't let that stop you from regular care.

Mind Update: SELF-CARE

Given all the focus on your baby, what have you done for *yourself* lately?

Every day, resolve to do one little thing that's just for you, just for fun, just because. Some ideas:

• Bring in fresh flowers (from your garden or the grocery).

• Serve yourself sparkling water or juice in a fancy wineglass.

• Buy a pair of silly socks.

• Binge-watch a guilty-pleasure show.

• Get a massage or ask someone to give you one.

• Eat some of your favorite chocolate.

• Try a new flavor of tea.

• Drive to a neighborhood you've never been in before, park, and walk.

• Buy a new lipstick.

• Meditate.

• Slip into a matinee and eat popcorn.

• Experiment with a bright scarf or pretty earrings to jazz up a basic maternity top.

• Download new music or ask your partner to craft you a pregnancy playlist.

• Paint your nails or get a manicure.

• Turn off all devices for a designated amount of "quiet time."

• Nap!

Biggest hopes and joys

Biggest fears and worries

Mighty is the force of motherhood.
It transforms all things by its vital heat.

GEORGE ELIOT

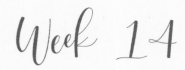

Week 14

Baby Update

Your baby's head is looking more and more proportional, mostly because the rest of the body is growing more rapidly now. This week, she is about 3-1/2 inches (8.9 cm) long and weighs around 1-1/2 ounces (42.5 g). A fuzzy layer of fine hair, called lanugo, is beginning to coat her entire body. Internally, the liver is starting to secrete bile, and the spleen is helping produce red blood cells. And, as the brain continues to mature, your baby can make different facial expressions.

Body Update: BREAKING OUT?

Many mothers-to-be experience bouts of acne, the likes of which they haven't seen since their teenage years. The same culprits are at fault now as were then—raging hormones, specifically estrogen and progesterone. Hormones may also cause heavier perspiration, causing heat rashes.

For acne-prone skin, use a gentle cleanser and remove any makeup completely before going to bed. Try switching to cosmetics and personal care products made for sensitive skin. Consult with your doctor about over-the-counter medications and avoid Retin-A, retinol, retinoic acid, isotretinoin and tazarotene, which have been linked to birth defects. Also on the smart-to-nix list: Tetracycline, salicylic acid, benzoyl peroxide. Cornstarch is helpful to keep heat rash-prone skin cool and dry.

You may also notice small, very fine red lines that seem to branch out under your skin on your face and neck. These are vascular spiders (spider nevi) and are completely harmless. There isn't much you can do about them, but they will disappear after childbirth.

Mind Update: FEELING SCATTERBRAINED?

Losing your keys. Forgetting a colleague's name. Walking upstairs to get . . . something, what was it again? Many pregnant women experience a sensation of memory loss and distraction. There is a lot on your mind, after all. Sleep disruptions, stress, excitement, and possibly hormonal changes can contribute to "momnesia."

Try these memory crutches:

• **Take notes in a special notebook or in your phone (or this journal).** Jot down everything from to-do lists to information that you would normally know off the top of your head (such as a shopping list).

• **Set reminder alerts.** Use them for paying bills, for appointments, even for meetings you're sure you'll remember. Set reminders or use apps that nudge you to stand up and stretch every hour or so.

• **Use visual aids.** Put your umbrella or sunglasses right by the door as memory joggers. Leave yourself post-it notes.

• **Add new key numbers to your contacts list.** Include anyone new to you in pregnancy, from your care provider and your favorite maternity store to home-delivery services.

• **Don't hide it—confide it.** Talk about any difficulty you're having with someone close to you. Other people might have suggestions that could help you stay organized, or be sources of "you're not crazy, you're pregnant" reassurance.

• **Give yourself a break.** Minimize multitasking and practice saying no.

DID YOU KNOW that weeks 14 to 18 are prime time to go on a babymoon, a pre-baby vacation getaway to reconnect with your partner? The fewest emergencies happen then, and you're most comfortable.

The best part of being pregnant so far

How I feel about my appearance right now

5 things I'll never do when I'm a mom

I ate two waffles, a banana, and cereal with blueberries.
And that was between my two breakfasts.

AMY POEHLER

Week 15

Baby Update

Your baby is about 4 inches (10.2 cm) long and weighs around 2 ounces (56.7 g). The limbs are getting longer now, especially the legs. His bones are starting to store calcium, or to ossify, which means that you could see his skeleton with an X-ray.

At the same time, your baby's ears are looking more "human" and the eyes are moving closer together. (They started out far on the sides of his head.) Vision is developing and even though the eyes remain closed, your baby can tell the difference between darkness and bright light around your belly.

Body Update: *BEATING DIETARY DOLDRUMS*

Getting tired of eating the same old things day after day? Spice up your diet with the occasional meal or snack that's unconventional for you. Your baby's taste buds are wiring up, so the flavors you eat—vanilla, garlic, anise, mint, carrots—have been shown to turn up in the amniotic fluid he's swallowing. Later he'll recognize these flavors in breast milk and be more likely to accept them as solids. Did someone say broccoli? Yum!

A few ideas:

• **Breakfast mixes.** Fill a tortilla with scrambled eggs, cheese, black beans, and vegetables or load an omelet with chopped kale, tomatoes, and herbs. Scoop fruit and Greek yogurt onto pancakes, waffles, or cereal.

• **Nuts for snacks.** They satisfy an urge to crunch and keep you full longer; try different kinds. Dip carrot sticks or apple slices in one of the many different nut butters, or stuff a date with some.

• **Multi-flavored pizza.** Experiment with vegetable toppings: salsa; grated bell peppers, carrots, or zucchini; roasted veggies; spinach; bean sprouts—almost anything goes.

• **Drink up nutrients.** Keep hydrated with fruit or green smoothies made with milk, yogurt (plain, Greek, or Icelandic), or milk alternatives (soy, almond, coconut, oat, cashew).

• **Savory snacks.** Try kale chips. They're easy to make, just toss a large bundle with 1 to 2 tablespoons of olive oil and a pinch of salt, and roast for 15 to 20 minutes at a low temperature, around 225 degrees. Or try roasted red-pepper hummus with carrot or pepper strips, edamame, roasted chickpeas, or popcorn dusted with rosemary and Parmesan, curry powder, or smoked paprika.

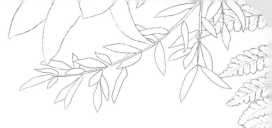

Mind Update: COMPARING NOTES

"You already felt your baby move?" "You mean you never felt sick or fat, ever?" As your pregnancy progresses, you may find yourself comparing yourself with other women. Talks and message boards can be good: you can share how you're feeling; ask one another questions; and share advice, support, and encouragement. But there's a potential downside, if judging yourself against a pregnant peer causes you to worry needlessly or feel like there's something "wrong" with you.

Remember that each pregnancy is different. Your weight gain, aches, and attitude toward medical care, nutrition, and other issues can be very different from someone else's (even your own mother's or your best friend's). And it's okay! Keep an open mind but trust your instincts and talk to your doctor if you have any concerns. To save on crazymaking, remind yourself there's only one You, only one Your Baby. (Okay, two or three if it's twins or triplets!)

DID YOU KNOW that soon after birth, babies show a preference for their mom's voice over another female's? They get used to hearing you in utero.

Nursery plans and ideas

Babymoon or pre-baby staycation plans

That's the strange thing about being a mother: Until you have a baby, you didn't even realize how much you were missing one.

Jodi Picoult

Week 16

Baby Update: WAS THAT IT?!

The amount of fine-tuning that's taken place in the last month is nothing short of miraculous. Your baby now measures about 4-1/2 inches (11.4 cm) and weighs around 3 ounces (85.1 g). She's just beginning a growth spurt. Her moves, from stretches to kicks to turns, get successively stronger as she gets bigger.

Body Update: WAS THAT THE BABY?!

Few things make you stop and take notice like the first time you think you feel your baby move inside you. Most women first become aware of this sensation, called "quickening," when they're about 16 to 22 weeks along. If you're slender, it can happen as early as 15 weeks.

The movement hits you just below the navel. It may feel like a soft nudge, a gas bubble or bubbles, or like being brushed from the inside by a flutter of wings. It's generally not for a few more weeks, when the baby grows and gets stronger, that you notice more decisive kicks and bumps. These "kicks," as they're collectively known, are intermittent, rather than constant. But sometimes so many movements will happen in quick succession that it'll seem like your little one is working out.

For many women, pregnancy becomes far more "real" once they've felt movement. Bear in mind that your partner may not be able to feel movements for a few more weeks—while you're experiencing them from the inside, others can feel them only from the outside.

Mind Update: *TOP MID-PREGNANCY WORRIES*

Every mom-to-be worries about something. Having a baby is such a huge unknown, it's only natural to play "what if" and "OMG!"

Here are a few frets that tend to cause more anxiety than they warrant:

• **Fear of miscarriage.** The weeks between when morning sickness ends but you haven't yet felt the baby move can be spooky: how do you know you're still pregnant? In the absence of bleeding or pain, everything's probably just fine. Confide your worries to your provider at your next visit, if you can't shake the feeling.

• **Fear of falls.** It's possible, because your center of gravity is changing. But even if you do tumble, you're unlikely to harm your baby. Maybe no more standing on stepladders to stash boxes in upper cupboards!

• **Fear of health problems in your baby.** Severe birth defects are rare in the overall population; testing can help ease worries. If you have a specific reason for concern, such as family history, talk to your doctor about additional genetic testing.

• **Fear of being a lousy mother.** The very fact that you're thinking about this subject says you want to do right by your baby—a sign of a very good parent! Whether you want to raise your child differently from how you were brought up, or just the same, looking at different role models and considering how you'll be are all cause for pats on the back, not anxiety attacks.

DID YOU KNOW that stretching pregnant skin tends toward dryness? Slather on the moisturizer and sunscreen.

When I felt my baby move

Where I was

How I knew

What it felt like

PEOPLE'S REACTIONS TO
THE NEWS ABOUT THE BABY

Parents

Siblings

Friends

Coworkers

Neighbors

Life is tough enough without having someone kick you from the inside.

Rita Rudner

Week 17

Baby Update

This week your baby is about 4-3/4 inches (12.1 cm) long and weighs about 4-1/2 ounces (127.6 g). Now that the body parts are in place, the body is starting to "fill out" and develop fat tissue.

The ears are positioned appropriately on the sides of the head, and hearing develops. Your voice and heartbeat are familiar sounds, so talk, sing, or read out loud! Also, starting now, your baby's umbilical cord is getting thicker and stronger (eventually it will be so tough, it'll take real effort to cut the cord after birth).

Body Update: COMFORT FOR LEG CRAMPS

Starting in your second trimester, you may feel sharp cramps in your legs. A "charley horse" muscle spasm in your foot, calf, or thigh is often felt when you're lying in bed or have been standing for a long time. These cramps may be the result of increasing pressure on your legs' nerves or a lack of calcium or magnesium.

To prevent cramps and find relief when they happen:

• **Stretch your calf muscles.** Do this by gently lunging (one foot forward) to a wall, keeping your feet flat on the floor and your back and the leg that's behind you straight (don't bounce).

• **Avoid standing or sitting in one place for too long.** If you must stand awhile, try wearing support/compression hose.

• **Set phone alerts that remind you to stand and stretch every hour.**

• **Add foods rich in calcium (yogurt), magnesium (quinoa), and/or potassium (bananas) to your diet.**

• **Extend your leg and stretch your foot (with toes pointed up) when you get a cramp.**

• **Softly massage the spasm or apply a heating pad to the affected area.**

Mind Update: BOND, BABY, BOND

You may feel even more connected to your baby from here on, what with hearing the heartbeat and feeling movement inside you. More ways to feel close:

• Make up a special baby name, just for now. (Hey there, Sprout!)

• Rub your belly as much as you like. It's a great connector that also relaxes you.

• Close your eyes and imagine your baby as a person, not just the alien-shaped tadpole you see in pregnancy apps and books. Picture taking a walk together. Imagine the warm sun, the heft of a snuggly baby in your arms. Nice, right?

DID YOU KNOW most parents want to know the baby's gender before birth? Gender reveal by ultrasound after 18 weeks is considered very reliable (unless you already found out via a blood test).

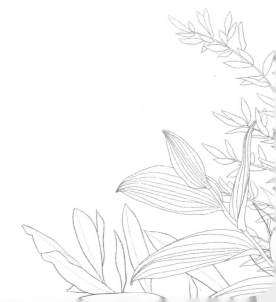

How I feel about having a boy

How I feel about having a girl

Pregnancy doubled her, birth halved her,
and motherhood turned her into Everywoman.

ERICA JONG

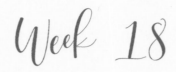
Week 18

Baby Update

Your baby has grown to about 5-1/2 inches (13.4 cm) and weighs around 5-1/2 ounces (156 g). The skeleton is made of rubbery cartilage, a "pre-bone" that gets harder and stronger in the coming weeks. Because your baby's growing bones will vampire yours to get the calcium they need, it's important to get enough calcium in your own diet.

Body Update: SEX AND THE NURSERY

Chances are your sexual desire is changing—for reasons that could include physical changes, a more positive or negative body image, your partner's attitudes, and the side effects of pregnancy like fatigue and discomfort, or other conditions. You may want sex more, surprising yourself at how much you daydream or fantasize about it. It may be easier to reach orgasm (due to hormones and increased blood flow). Many pregnant women say their desire peaks during the second trimester. Alternatively, you may want it less, dreading even the suggestion of foreplay.

Whichever way you're ebbing and flowing (and it can change daily), talking with your partner about how you're each feeling can keep you close—especially if you can keep a sense of humor about working around your growing bump. Experiment with different positions as you expand. (Avoid lying flat on your back.) Just don't worry about your baby. He or she will be perfectly fine. Sex can't trigger miscarriage or labor.

Mind Update: PREGNANT DREAMS

Have you been surprised by a particularly vivid, strange dream or frightening nightmare lately? Some pregnant women dream of their baby in bewildering forms (a piglet? a loaf of bread?). A common dream is that you forget to care for your child. And no, they're not omens that you're going to be a terrible mother! Your mind is trying to cope with a lot of information as you undergo significant physical and emotional changes and as you anticipate the lifestyle changes coming your way. It's logical that your mind would work overtime then, sorting things out as you sleep.

One bright side: At this point in pregnancy, you're more likely to wake up during REM sleep (light, or dream sleep). That makes it more likely you can remember your dreams. They can be interesting to puzzle over. For example, a dream about losing the baby may help you deal with a fear of miscarriage that you would rather ignore when you're awake. You may dream about your competence (or imagined lack thereof) in taking care of a literal "bun in the oven." Your protective maternal instinct may also creep up in dreams in which you and your baby are threatened (as during a crime or accident).

There are no for-sure answers for what's behind your dreams. If they're stressing you, try doing a little research in a book about dreams and their meanings. Sometimes a therapist, if you are seeing one, can help you explore interpretations. Compare dreams with your partner—who may be having some wild ones, too.

Dreams

*The best thing I heard today was a pregnant woman arguing with her partner
and she said, "I have two brains and you have one."*

AUTHOR UNKNOWN

Week 19

Most mothers-to-be have felt the baby move by now; if you haven't, give it a few more weeks.

Baby Update

Although your baby still weighs less than a pound, she's getting heavier as fat stores increase. Your baby measures about 6 inches (15.2 cm) this week. Hair appears, on the head and as eyebrows and eyelashes. And even though they won't make their debut until years from now, permanent teeth buds are developing under the gums, behind the milk teeth (baby teeth) buds. Also, this week, your baby's brain is assigning specific areas to support each of the five senses.

Brace yourself for ever more gymnastics. Beyond kicks and stretches, your baby may flip upside down, twist and roll from side to side. Later in pregnancy, though, these movements won't be so dramatic because there will be less space in the uterus for them.

Body Update: SLEEPUS INTERRUPTUS?

Good night to getting a good night's rest! You might find you have to keep getting up to use the bathroom. Fetal movements, an inability to get comfortable, and a racing mind can all add to sleep trouble.

Ten tips:

• **Keep it routine.** Try to go to bed and get up at about the same time every day and night. Skip or shorten naps by day.

• **Make your room sleep friendly.** Lose the TV set, turn off all devices, keep the room dark and free of distractions.

• **Check your caffeine intake and cut back.** Good rule of thumb: No tea or coffee after about noon.

• **Quit bright screens a couple of hours before bed.** Or use a setting or app that blocks or filters blue/green wavelengths, which can interfere with your circadian rhythm.

• **Try keeping the room on the cool side.** Temperatures between 65 to 70 degrees F (18 to 20 C) encourage the body to sleep.

• **Get plenty of exercise and fresh air by day.** Even sitting outdoors can help.

• **Consume as few liquids as possible after dinner.** You'll be less likely to have to get up and disrupt your sleep.

• **Try deep breathing or mindfulness to help you drift off.** Count breaths—or sheep.

• **Stop nighttime ruminating.** Think about something happy, like your baby's first birthday party. Corny, but it works.

• **Add more pillows as needed.** Get yourself comfortable from now until your due date.

Mind Update: INVOLVING YOUR PARTNER

You become the center of attention as family and friends—and even strangers—rally around the "visible" baby you're carrying.

Help your partner avoid feeling left out:

• Go together to your prenatal appointments.

• Encourage your partner to bond by feeling your belly for kicks and talking or reading to your baby.

• Talk together about your hopes for your baby, guess what your baby might be like, and reminisce about your own childhoods.

• Plan your baby registry together and split nursery-making chores. (Hello, crib assembly!)

• Involve your partner in all major decisions—from baby names to medical care.

• Exercise together.

• Attend childbirth, breastfeeding, and other classes together.

• Compare your answers to the prompts in this book. What's similar? What's different?

A To-Do list for my partner

(THANKS, DEAR!)

Waiting for this baby is like picking up someone from the airport, but you don't know who they are or what time their flight comes in.

AUTHOR UNKNOWN

Week 20

Congratulations! You're halfway to motherhood!

Baby Update: THE MIDWAY POINT!

Now that your baby has stretched his legs out a bit, his length is measured from the crown of his head to his heel. The average fetus is now about 9-1/2 inches (24.1 cm) long and weighs around 9 ounces (255 g). A smooth white layer of *vernix caseosa*, a natural substance that's like baby's first moisturizer, covers your baby's body to protect the skin while living submerged in its watery crib.

Also around this time, he starts converting waste into dark and sticky meconium, a "pre-poop" that will probably test your skills as a baby wiper during your first few diaper changes.

Body Update: BACK CARE

One side effect of your growing baby and expanding uterus is a shifting center of gravity. Your back works extra hard to provide support—no wonder it aches sometimes!

Protect your spine and back muscles by being especially careful to use good posture. Follow these tips:

• **When you walk:** Keep your shoulders back and your spine as straight as possible. Most women find the most comfort wearing low, supportive heels (1/2 inch to 2 inches, or 1 to 5 cm), rather than complete flats or skyscrapers.

• **When you sit:** Sit with your back straight and legs uncrossed. If you must stand or sit in one place for long periods, such as at work, elevate one of your feet on a low stool. At a desk, sit directly facing your paperwork or computer. Try using a pillow to support the small of your back.

• **When you sleep:** Don't lie flat on your back. Make sure you have a firm mattress; if yours is more than 10 years old, this is a great excuse to upgrade.

• **When you lift:** Stand with your feet apart, bend at your knees (not your waist), and let your arms and legs do the work.

Relieve your backache with these feel-good exercises:

• **Stand with your back and shoulders against a wall.** Tighten your abdominal muscles and gently pull your stomach in and tilt the pelvis upward. Hold that position for about 5 seconds. Return to the starting position. This "pelvic tilt" can also be done lying on the floor with your legs partly bent, feet flat on the floor.

• **Get on all fours, with your hands flat on the floor and your back straight.** Tighten your abdominal muscles and gently curl your lower back upward, like a cat. Hold that position for about 5 seconds. Return to the starting position.

• **Put your hands on your shoulders and roll your elbows front to back.**

Mind Update: FEELING LESS THAN PERFECT

So maybe you weigh more than you expected you would by this point in pregnancy. Or you already have stretch marks. Or you're sick of everyone yammering about the baby and how excited you must be—and you feel guilty for feeling this way. Say you don't know how you can possibly make it all the way until your due date. Point is, everybody can find something about her pregnancy that's off-key, not quite what she expected.

What to do about it?

• **Repeat over and over:** There is no such thing as a perfect pregnancy. Your motto now more than ever: "Me B Me."

• **Go with the flow.** Some days are smooth, others feel like you're shooting the rapids. Consider it preparation for motherhood.

• **Go ahead and grouse.** Some women get stretch marks now, some get colicky babies later. The universe isn't fair, and neither is pregnancy. Though you can't have wine, you're entitled to whine.

DID YOU KNOW that, for some women, significant fatigue continues well into the second trimester?

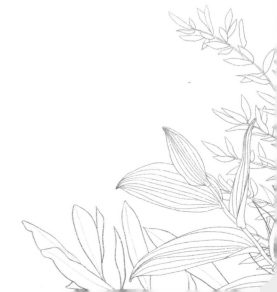

What makes me happy

I felt like a part of a huge happy community of women. Even in New York City, strangers talked to me as if I were their cousin.

RISA MAY

ULTRASOUND IMAGES

Week 21

Baby Update: HELLO, BIG BOY OR GIRL!

Your baby is now about 10 inches (25.4 cm) long and weighs around 10-1/2 ounces (297.7 g). The digestive system is maturing; while swallowing amniotic fluid, your baby absorbs some water and nutrients from it. If your baby is a girl, your future grandchildren are already in place in the form of her eggs!

Your baby is getting plenty of exercise inside of you and you might wonder if your baby is a night owl based on its "schedule." The truth is: your movement throughout the day likely rocks your baby to sleep, so when you're ready for bed, your baby's raring to go. It has a circadian rhythm now, just not exactly yours.

Body Update: WEIGHT GAIN

It's natural to wonder about your weight gain. The "typical" pregnancy should result in a weight gain of 25 to 35 pounds (about 12 to 16 kg). But our culture is so conditioned to think negatively about weight gain in general, it can be hard for a woman to keep perspective. Baby weight is good weight! Your baby can't thrive without it!

After the initial 3 or 4 pounds (1.4 or 1.8 kg) gained in the first trimester, most women add about a pound (454 g) a week during the last two trimesters. That's only a very rough rule of thumb—not a prescription. Your provider will monitor your weight to make sure it's healthy for you and your baby.

Here's a breakdown of how the weight of a typical 30-pound (13.6-kg) gain is distributed:

Baby = 7-1/2 pounds (3.4 kg)   **Placenta** = 1-1/2 pounds (680 g)

Amniotic fluid = 2 pounds (907 g)   **Uterus** = 2 pounds (907 g)

Breasts = 2 pounds (907 g)   **Body stores** = 7 pounds (3.18 kg)

Blood = 4 pounds (1.8 kg)   **Other body fluids** = 4 pounds (1.8 kg)

Your doctor may encourage you to gain less if you were overweight pre-pregnancy, or more if you were underweight.

Mind Update: WHAT TO WEAR

For a while, you can pop open a button on your jeans or pop on a loose popover top. But eventually your popping bump will start screaming, "Get me something that fits!"

When building your new wardrobe:

• **Choose basic pieces that you can mix and match.** Leggings and yoga pants (maternity-specific or not) are even more of a godsend in pregnancy.

• **Give yourself some room to grow.** Pick clothes that fit well now but have some room. Believe it or not it's possible to outgrow a roomy maternity top before you deliver. Stretch fabrics and adjustable features, like a tie on the back of a blouse, help.

• **Consider the dress.** They're comfy and handy to have on hand for a special event. Buy a solid color and vary your look with scarves or other accessories.

• **Browse your partner's wardrobe.** A man's plain white button-down shirt makes a good shirt or jacket.

• **Borrow from friends and family, or check consignment shops.** A new mother can be a pregnant woman's best friend.

• **Update your underwear drawer too, as needed**. It's not just bras that keep growing; you might feel better in roomier undies.

• **Help keep your body temperature comfortable by choosing natural fibers.** Say yes to cotton, linen, silk, merino, and lightweight fabrics that you can layer.

• **Avoid overbuying.** You want enough to feel comfortable but these aren't "forever" clothes. Some shirts and bras designed for nursing mothers can do double duty now and later.

DID YOU KNOW that there's no standard "look" for a pregnant belly? Some women carry higher or lower than others, stick out more in front, or barely seem to show at all by mid-pregnancy.

How I'm dressing my bump

I'm pregnant, which means I'm sober, swollen, and hungry. Approach with caution.

AUTHOR UNKNOWN

Week 22

Baby Update

This week your baby is about 10-1/2 inches (26.7 cm) long and weighs around 13 ounces (368.5 g). Despite the padding your baby is acquiring, filling out occurs slowly, so it still looks a little wrinkly. The skin is so thin that you can see a network of blood vessels underneath it. But facial features are more visible now, including minuscule lips, fully formed eyelids, and fine eyebrows. Some parents are surprised at how distinctive the features may appear on an ultrasound. Her eyes are also fully formed, though pigment has yet to color them. Also around this time, your baby's liver and pancreas continue to develop.

Body Update: KICK COUNTS

Your baby's athletics are more than entertaining. They provide reassurance that all's well. (A baby who has stopped moving for long periods may be asleep, or, much less likely, may have become tangled in the umbilical cord or have another problem.) For this reason, doctors recommend that expectant mothers monitor their baby's movements periodically through the day. You don't have to be obsessive about this. It's simply a matter of pausing to pay attention.

Your doctor or midwife may suggest her preferred method. A simple way: Choose a starting time and begin counting movements. Once you reach 10, note the time and calculate the number of minutes it took. If you don't reach 10 in an hour, have a snack or a glass of juice and try again.

If you have any concerns about your baby's activity or you notice fewer than 10 movements in an hour (after eating a snack or drinking juice), notify your provider. There are simple noninvasive tests that can be done in the office to stimulate movement and further assess fetal well-being.

Mind Update: *HANDLING UNWANTED ADVICE*

A swelling belly is like a magnet for advice givers, drawing them to you with ever so helpful tips, suggestions, and judgments. Or not so helpful. "Your heels are too high," "That coffee is bad for your baby," "I saw a great device you need," "Did you know that . . ."

How to cope?

• **First, consider the source.** Women who have had children before you can be founts of knowledge, so don't dismiss all the advice automatically. Sometimes someone else's experience can save you time or money. Remember most people are just trying to help.

• **Forgive their bloopers.** In their excitement over your condition, friends and strangers alike tend to overstep boundaries without realizing it, saying things to a pregnant woman (like, "Don't you know doughnuts have little nutritional value?") that they'd never dream of saying to someone who wasn't pregnant. Chalk it up to good intentions. It's their way of showing that they care (even if they are being busybodies).

• **Politely ignore the dubious and the dangerous.** Told about an herb potion sure to vanquish stretch marks or an exercise regimen you aren't sure about? Say something benign like, "That sounds interesting; I'll ask my doctor." If your persistent counselor asks later why you haven't been doing what they suggested, blame your obstetrician: "My doctor would rather I not try that."

• **Exit when you've had enough.** When the advice expands from a comment to a tirade, offer a cool, "Thanks for your interest," and change the subject. Ask for opinions about something benign like nursery decorations. Or excuse yourself to use the restroom (yet again!).

DID YOU KNOW that some tattoos can stretch or fade in pregnancy?

What feels new this week

My favorite things about being pregnant

Head-to-toe inventory of what's different about my body

Pregnant women! They had that weird frisson, an aura of magic that combined awkwardly with an earthy sense of duty. Mundane, because they were nothing unique on the suburban streets; ethereal because their attention was ever somewhere else. Whatever you said was trivial. And they had that preciousness which they imposed wherever they went, compelling attention, constantly reminding you that they carried the future inside, its contours already drawn, but veiled, private, an inner secret.

RUTH MORGAN

Week 23

Baby Update

About 11 inches (27.9 cm) long, your baby now weighs a grand total of 1 pound (453.6 g). As he gains weight and moves around, muscles are being strengthened. Air sacs (alveoli) and blood vessels are also developing in the lungs just about now, getting your baby ready to breathe. However, the lungs would still be too immature to do the job on their own and if he were born now, mechanical support would be required. Even though he won't breathe until birth, he "practices" by inhaling and exhaling amniotic fluid.

The hearing is also improving. Your baby may begin to grow accustomed to the usual loud noises produced by your body or around your home. Some researchers believe that listening to music calms a fetus. (It's even been said that babies in the womb who hear a dog bark will be less likely to be spooked as newborns.)

Body Update: *QUICK NUTRITIOUS SNACK IDEAS*

Ransacking the cupboards looking for something to eat? Many women prefer small mini-meals as their digestive system begins to be rearranged by the expanding uterus.

Good-for-you snacks help satisfy nibbles:

• Add nut butter to other foods, such as apple slices, rice cakes, or celery sticks.

• Make hummus or bean dip for your veggies.

• Mix fresh or canned fruit (in its own juice, not syrup) with cottage cheese or yogurt.

• Stock up on healthy finger foods that you can eat on the go, such as seedless grapes, frozen grapes, air-popped popcorn.

• Make a grain bowl from quinoa, farro, or another grain, mixed with leftover roasted vegetables and chopped greens.

• Make a trail mix of your favorite dried fruits, seeds, nuts, and yeah, some chocolate chips.

• Treat yourself to exotic fruits you don't usually buy, like mangoes, papayas, and kiwi.

• Microwave a sweet potato and top with cheese and black beans.

• Make a roll-up. Spread cream cheese and/or mashed avocado on a tortilla or flat bread. Pile on thin slices of vegetables, such as cucumber, tomato, and onion, and roll it up. Chop the roll into bite-size segments.

Mind Update: REACH OUT AND (DON'T) TOUCH ME!

You may notice an interesting phenomenon: The more you show, the more inclined people are to want to rub your belly! It is hard to ignore, after all. Some women aren't bothered by playing lucky Buddha, and even welcome the chance to share their pregnancy in this way. Others grow irritated or take offense at having their personal boundary crossed. The touchers rarely see themselves as being rude or intrusive. They imagine themselves touching not you but the baby.

If you've had enough, it's your pregnant prerogative to say, "Please don't do that," or "Please stop; it's making me uncomfortable." The belly-patter won't know if you're referring to your feelings or your physical state, and if upsetting you doesn't motivate him or her to cease and desist, the idea of doing anything that might be bad for the baby usually does the trick.

Try deflecting the situation with humor: "Look, but don't touch." Or "You can pat mine if I can pat yours."

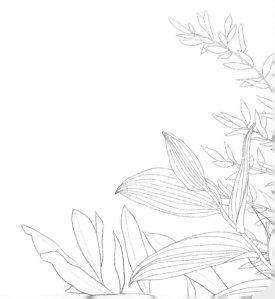

Childhood memories I'd like to repeat for my baby

My partner's childhood memories we'd like to repeat

In the middle of a boring meeting at work or a meaningless argument, you feel your baby squirming inside you and the sensation takes you away. It's your own secret communication.

Heather Moors Johnson, Parents.com

Week 24

Most women have a glucose screening between 24 and 28 weeks to screen for the need for further testing for gestational diabetes.

Baby Update

This week your baby is almost at the 1-foot (30.5 cm) mark. Average weight: about 1-1/4 pounds (567 g). It's a time of "more of the same." The brain continues to develop. By birth, it will still be only partially "online" and require the first 3 years of life to wire up to its full processing of sight, sound, and other stimuli. The lungs are branching out and developing cells to make surfactant, which helps the air sacs inflate. His taste buds are also under development now.

Your baby still moves quite a bit, even though the amniotic sac is becoming somewhat of a tight fit. The amniotic fluid allows him to move safely and relatively easily.

Body Update: BELLY BASICS

As the skin on your abdomen stretches, you may begin to feel some itchiness. This is normal. Try not to scratch or you could make the dry skin feel even worse. Instead, try using some moisturizer or shea butter (applying it as soon as you step out of the shower). Avoid soap that dries your skin.

At the same time, you may start to notice thin pink, reddish, or purplish lines branching out across your abdomen. Although some creams and lotions promise to prevent or reduce the appearance of stretch marks, none have been proven to work. You may be able to prevent them somewhat by gaining weight gradually and within your recommended range. These marks will likely fade significantly or disappear completely on their own with time. If they last longer than six months postpartum and they bother you very much, talk to a dermatologist.

Mind Update: OLD WIVES' TALES

"Young wives" tell them, too. Old wives' tales are superstitious beliefs rooted in folklore, and pregnancy is rife with them. They can be fun to think about, if you don't take them too seriously. Or you can just safely ignore them—no matter how persistently a nosy lady in the supermarket repeats them.

Here are some golden oldies that are NOT true:

If you have a lot of heartburn, your baby will have a lot of hair. Acne signals a girl because she's stealing your beauty. Eating strawberries causes reddish birthmarks. Cutting your hair during pregnancy robs a fetus of its energy. If you go swimming you might drown the baby. Craving sweets means a boy; craving sours means a girl. Worrying too much in pregnancy will give you a boy. Boys are more active in the womb. Don't lift your arms above your head or you might cause a knot in the umbilical cord. Young children can predict your baby's gender. Carrying high means it's a girl; carrying low indicates a boy.

Here are a few pregnancy clichés that ARE true:

• **Pregnancy makes your feet grow.** Thank the hormone relaxin, which loosens all your joints in order to prepare your pelvis for delivery.

• **Labor often starts at night.** The production of oxytocin, a hormone that causes contractions, peaks in the evening.

• **Second babies are easier to deliver.** Second labors tend to be shorter on average than first labors because the muscles involved have already stretched some and your pelvic bones may be wider. However, if your firstborn was delivered by C-section, your next labor is more likely to progress like a first-timer's.

DID YOU KNOW that babies nap in utero?

When I listen to my body, it says . . .

10 things I plan to do differently from my parents

You are the bows from which your children as living arrows are sent forth.

KAHLIL GIBRAN

Week 25

Baby Update

Your baby is about 12-1/2 inches (31.8 cm) long and weighs around 1-1/2 pounds (680.4 g). She is slowly on the way to looking more like a cuddly newborn as her body bulks up with more baby fat. But more important, growing a good layer of fat tissue will help her regulate her own body temperature outside the womb and will provide energy. By now, your baby's hair might also have a certain color and texture, but these could change after birth and she might lose this first head of hair altogether.

Body Update: *READYING FOR CHILDBIRTH*

A simple way to prepare your body to support and, later, deliver your baby is to strengthen your pelvic floor muscles.

There are several methods:

• **Kegels.** These exercises are very easy and nobody can tell you're doing them. Just tighten up as if you were stopping a flow of urine and hold for 5 seconds. (But don't practice while you're urinating, as this can cause an infection.) Start with 5 Kegels, 5 times a day and work up to 10 Kegels, 10 times a day. You can also later increase the number of seconds you hold to 10. A more advanced technique is to contract your muscles in "steps" and then slowly relax one step at a time (this is sometimes called the elevator Kegel).

• **Tailor sitting.** This exercise prepares your groin and upper legs. Get into position as if you were going to sit cross-legged on the floor. Instead of crossing your ankles, though, pull one ankle into your body and pull the other one just in front of it. Alternately, you can bring the soles of your feet together. Then lean forward slightly so your knees almost reach the floor. Hold for as long as you can without straining (try for 2 minutes at a time, several times a day).

• **Squats.** These help widen your pelvic opening and work your legs. With your hands on a piece of furniture for support, stand with your feet apart (a little wider than your hips) and your toes pointed slightly outward. Bend your legs, keeping your back straight and your heels on the floor, and lower into a sitting position. Exhale as you stretch your legs to return to standing position.

Mind Update: STORIES YOU'D RATHER NOT HEAR

Everybody, it seems, has a birth story to share—their own or some long saga that happened to their cousin, sister, or celebrity. Hearing such stories can help you prepare for your own experience. Some stories can spook you.

Here are some tips for dealing with unwanted stories:

• **Nip it.** Before the person gets too far, smile and say, "This isn't another horror story, is it? Please don't harsh my happy!"

• **Disrupt it.** Politely cut off the storyteller with, "Thanks, but I'd really rather not talk about this." Be honest about your nerves. You'll likely hear some reassurance instead. If the stories continue, excuse yourself to use the bathroom.

• **Recruit your partner or a friend to be your advocate.** Ask them to let people know you'd rather not hear about bad experiences. (This is useful at baby showers.)

• **Get it out of your system.** After hearing a story you wish you hadn't, debrief with a compassionate friend or your partner, or by writing about it.

• **Counteract it.** Seek out positive stories from people who you know had wonderful deliveries. In real life, the great births far outweigh the unhappy ones.

DID YOU KNOW that while some swelling of the face or ankles is to be expected, puffiness can also be a sign of *preeclampsia* (see page 150)? That's why you should pay attention to what seems normal for YOU, and report changes.

3 things I'm grateful for

Why would anyone trust me with a baby?

SUZANNE FINNAMORE, *THE ZYGOTE CHRONICLES*

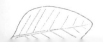

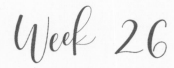

Week 26

You're now entering the zone of viability for your baby to likely survive outside the womb without lasting troubles (still with lots of help). Every extra week now is ginormous in terms of benefit to your baby's health.

Baby Update

From here on out, your baby is gaining weight steadily in preparation for life outside the womb. Your baby is nearing the 2-pound (907.2 g) mark, averaging 13-1/2 inches (34.3 cm) long. Repeated poke-poke-pokes might be hiccups, a common reflex that helps practice for later breathing.

Body Update: MEASURING UP?

If you measure "off" for your dates, ask a lot of questions. Your fundal height is usually the same now in centimeters as your weeks of pregnancy (so, 25 cm this week). When your measurement is larger or smaller than expected for your gestational age, there can be lots of reasons that have nothing to do with your due date.

These can include:

• **If you're measuring large:** your individual size and shape (like having more slack abdominal muscles), the baby's position, twins or other multiples, gestational diabetes, or a big baby.

• **If you're measuring small:** your individual size or shape, a small but fine baby, growth issues with the placenta or baby, a health issue for you (like smoking or infection).

An ultrasound and other monitoring can help uncover the reason. But it won't make your due date any more predictable. Don't get too attached to your due date . . . it's just a numbers game! Even if you're sure of the exact moment of conception, there's still a five-week window (weeks 37 to 41) during which your baby can turn up and be considered healthy and full term.

Mind Update: CHOOSING A CHILDBIRTH CLASS

Now is a good time to start considering a childbirth class, which is best taken in the early to mid-last trimester. Sometimes classes fill up quickly, and you want to make sure you get a spot in a class scheduled to finish at least three weeks before your due date. To find classes, ask trusted friends, your doctor or midwife, and nurses. Look online for what's nearby. There may be classes offered at the place where you plan to give birth.

More tips for picking a class:

• **Ask for a description of what the class will cover.** Vaginal and cesarean births? (Most women don't know which they'll have; be prepared for either.) Drug-free and drug-assisted labor? Any postpartum recovery and newborn care information?

• **Find out what kinds of relaxation and pain-management techniques are taught.** Ask about the level of coach involvement.

• **Read up or ask about the methods taught, such as Lamaze, HypnoBirthing, Alexander, and Bradley.** Some teach a variety of breathing and relaxation techniques.

• **Ask about class size.** You get more personal attention in a smaller class.

• **Consider the schedule.** An all-in-one-day course is convenient but presents an awful lot of ground to absorb. A six-or-more week course requires a greater time commitment but can aid retention.

• **Consider the background and qualifications of potential class instructors.** Personal fit is important, too. It helps if you "click" with your instructor.

• **Consider YouTube or other online video classes in a pinch.** Though a live instructor can answer questions best, some prep is better than no prep.

DID YOU KNOW that your baby's brain weight triples in the last 13 weeks of pregnancy?

Childbirth class information

Questions about childbirth

That moment when your belly unknowingly becomes your table.

Ciara

Week 27

Baby Update

Your baby is now about 14 inches (35.6 cm) long and weighs around 2 pounds (907 g) and is beginning to open and close his eyes around this time. The retina, which receives light information, is starting to function, and the brain is maturing and able to interpret this information. A baby can not only recognize light shining through your belly, but also turn his eyes toward it.

Your baby has probably adopted a consistent sleep/wake cycle, which may be the reverse of your own. (Your movements by day lull your baby to sleep. Many parents must teach their newborns the difference between night and day partly because of this.)

Body Update: KEEP MOVING!

Reevaluate your exercise program to make sure it still suits your energy level, sense of balance, and comfort level.

If you're looking for some fresh ideas, try these:

• **Hit the pool.** Swimming is generally a safe activity during pregnancy (and it's great to feel weightless for a while).

• **Try prenatal Pilates or yoga videos, as long as your doctor says it's okay.**

• **Join a prenatal exercise class approved by your doctor.**

• **Shop for baby furniture, put it together, and start decorating the nursery.** This all takes energy.

• **Clean house.** Once the baby comes, household chores will likely fall to the bottom of your priority list, so take advantage and get organized now.

• **Spend some time outdoors.** Try taking a 30-minute walk every day.

• **Alternate activity with rest.**

Mind Update: *CHOOSING YOUR BABY'S DOCTOR*

It may seem early, but you'll want to have a doctor for your baby in place before you deliver, and the selection process can take a little time. First, you'll need to decide if you prefer a pediatrician (a physician who has specialized in the care of babies and children) or a family doctor (a physician who could take care of your entire family, including your child as an adolescent).

Poll family, friends, and your obstetric care provider for recommendations. Ask about the doctor's sensitivity to different views, friendliness, and responsiveness to questions. Check whether certain doctors are covered under your health insurance. Convenience to you (distance from your home and parking options) and after-hours availability (because children always seem to get sick at night and on weekends) are also important considerations. Once you have a list of candidates, schedule some interview appointments to get to know the doctors better. Ideally you and your partner should both attend. Some doctors may charge for this visit.

Here are some topics to cover:

• **Find out about availability:** What are the doctor's hours? What happens if you have a question after hours? What about emergencies? Does the doctor have privileges at the nearest children's hospital? If the doctor is part of a group, can your baby always see the same doctor?

• **Ask about how the doctor's office treats sick children.** How soon can your child be seen if he gets sick? Are sick children kept waiting in a separate area?

• **Discuss views on issues that are important to you.** Support for breastfeeding or bottle-feeding, immunizations, and circumcision.

• **Chat about the doctor's background and experience.** Any subspecialties? Is he or she a parent?

• **Ask when the doctor would first see your baby and what would happen during the visit.**

First impressions of the doctor, his office, and his staff count: Did you feel comfortable? Did you find it easy to talk to everyone and ask questions? Were the doctor's explanations clear and thorough? Were you kept waiting long before the appointment? Did the office seem clean and organized? You'll be spending a lot of time (and money) with this professional in the coming years. Take your time and make a selection you feel good about.

Baby doctor notes: Questions to ask

If every body is a work of art, what kind of masterpiece is a mother's body?
One that sacrifices so much of itself to create, harbor, and give birth to new life?

ANNIE RENEAU

How I feel heading into the last trimester

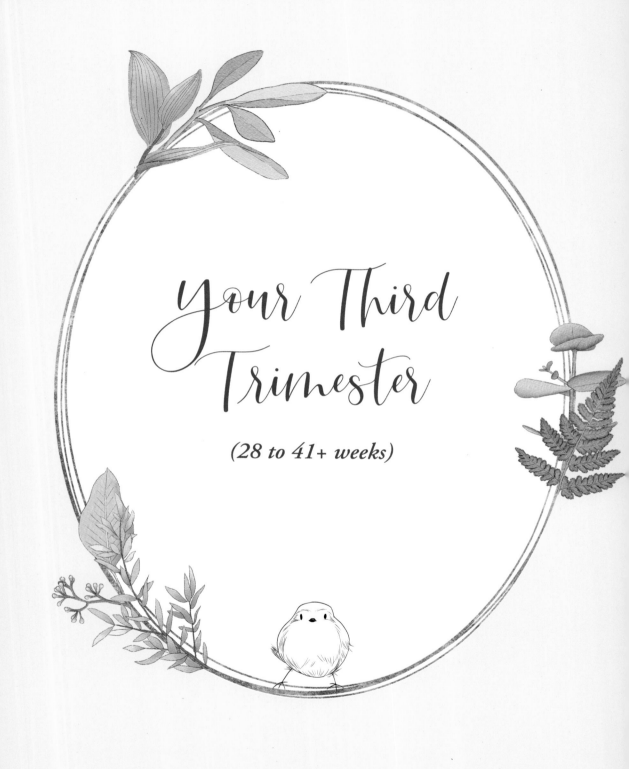

Your Third
Trimester

(28 to 41+ weeks)

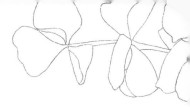

The Homestretch

The last trimester of pregnancy is one of the wildest times of your life because You Are Definitely About to Have a Baby! You look it. You feel it. Strangers can tell. The more frequent doctor visits say so, too.

It's a time of ready-to-go excitement and plodding fatigue. Of thinking about tiny baby clothes and barely being able to button your own. Of time passing maddeningly slowly and yet there not being enough time to get everything done.

Take advantage of these weeks to make final plans and preparations for motherhood. At work, make sure you've talked to your human resources contact about paperwork, insurance, and the like. You should also evaluate your post-birth work plans and plan your maternity leave or quit date with your supervisor. At home, you'll want to start assembling the furniture, gear, and clothing your baby will need, or, if this goes against cultural or religious conventions for you, at least make lists of what you'll need and arrangements for their delivery later. With your partner, compare notes about feelings during these countdown weeks and share one another's expectations about baby care and finding time for your relationship after you become parents.

Think help, too! What do you need to know or do to prepare yourself for labor and delivery, for breastfeeding, for baby care? Whom can you turn to for advice? Call your provider whenever you're in doubt about anything. And leave time to dream a little, too.

The last three months of pregnancy are a time for wondering, wishing, and—yes—waiting.

Third Trimester

DOS AND DON'TS

DO . . .

• **Expect to gain about 1 to 1-1/2 pounds (454 to 680 g) a week this trimester.** Your baby adds the most body weight now in preparation for life outside the womb.

• **Expect more face time with your provider.** Check-ups increase to every two weeks soon, then weekly. Keep jotting down your questions so you remember them; pregnancy brain fog really is a thing!

• **Eat lots of small meals.** Your nutritional needs are the same as in mid-pregnancy, but, as your uterus compresses your stomach, you may feel more comfortable if you consume less at each sitting.

• **Drink lots of water.** Staying well-hydrated enhances blood production, wards off constipation, and may help you avoid premature contractions. Carry an athletic bottle around with you so you can sip all day.

• **Continue taking your prenatal vitamins.** Don't forget to refill your prescription before the bottle is empty.

• **Start using stork/new-mom parking spaces.** You qualify.

• **Keep moving.** Exercise makes you feel better and sleep better, and helps your body to prepare, overall, for delivery.

• **Rehearse your delivery.** Know how to reach your partner at all times by the ninth month and have a backup plan for getting to the birth center. Take care of hospital-admittance paperwork ahead of time. And be sure you know directions to the place where you'll deliver and where to check in once you get there.

• **Take a childbirth class that will end at least 3 weeks before your due date.** That way, you're sure to finish it.

• **Continue doing kick counts to monitor your baby's well-being.** (See page 98.) Pay attention to how the kicks seem to change as your pregnancy progresses. As space grows tight, they may feel less broad and more isolated and even sharp.

• **Read up on breastfeeding and parenting techniques while you have the time.** In the first busy weeks of parenthood you're likely to have less time.

DON'T . . .

• **Don't be too impatient.** Use these weeks to savor the relative freedom of childlessness and reinforce your relationship while it's "just the two of you" (if this is your first child).

• **Don't skip the seat belt because it's uncomfortable.** You're buckling up for two.

• **Don't overdo it.** Listen to your body, which may be signaling a need for increased rest as your pregnancy progresses. Aim for a balance between moving and relaxing.

• **Don't use step stools or ladders, or otherwise put yourself at risk for falls.** Your altered sense of balance is already a risk factor.

• **Don't ignore bothersome symptoms or hesitate to call and ask your provider about anything.** You're likely to encounter more new weird symptoms as you get bigger, so questions are expected.

• **Don't bother with fetal keepsake videos.** The FDA "strongly discourages" them unless for medical purposes, even though ultrasounds aren't found to carry risks. (There just aren't enough studies yet.)

• **Don't shy from hard thoughts.** It's hard to ignore the physical reality of being pregnant, but some women also avoid talking about or thinking about the baby growing inside them. If this sounds familiar, explore what's behind this denial. Is it fear of how your life will change? Fear you won't be taken as seriously at work? Ambivalence about motherhood? There are no "bad" thoughts; it's only "bad" to ignore feelings, whatever form they take. Use this journal to write about your worries as well as your wishes.

• **Don't call yourself "fat."** What you—and everyone who looks at you—are seeing is the miracle of new life in progress.

When I listen to my body, it says . . .

When I listen to my heart, it says . . .

Questions for my provider

In pregnancy, there are two bodies, one inside the other. Two people live under one skin.
When so much of life is dedicated to maintaining our integrity as distinct beings,
this bodily tandem is an uncanny fact.

JOAN RAPHAEL-LEFF

Week 28

If your blood is Rh negative, you'll probably receive a shot of RhoGAM by this week to prevent you from being sensitized if your baby's Rh-positive blood mixes with yours.

Baby Update

During the second trimester, the growth rate of an individual fetus begins to vary somewhat based on genetics and other factors. By this week, the average baby measures a little over 14 inches (35.6 cm) and weighs around 2-1/4 pounds (1.02 kg). She continues to look fuller as fat tissue is added. The skin is still thin and shiny pink, but begins to appear more opaque.

One thing you might notice: fetal hiccups. They feel like repetitive blips and happen more often now as your baby's respiratory system continues to develop.

Body Update: THE SKIN YOU'RE IN

The hormonal shifts of pregnancy can have some surprising effects on your skin. Not all women experience every change, depending on heredity, pigment, and other individual factors. Most of these skin changes revert to normal after delivery.

Here are a few surprising—but completely harmless—changes you may notice:

• **A single thin, dark line stretching down your abdomen from the navel to the pubic bone.** This is called the *linea nigra*. Believe it or not, this line was there even before you got pregnant, but it normally matches your skin shade. It fades after delivery, but this can take several months.

• **Patches of discolored skin.** Called *chloasma*, this is an effect of your increased vulnerability to sun, especially on your face. The patches tend to look tan on light skin and lighter on darker skin. Take extra care to avoid overexposure and always use sunscreen when you go outdoors. (Chloasma can show up even when you stay inside, however.)

• **Darker freckles or moles.** Scars and birthmarks can darken, too. Again, blame hormones and sun exposure. Do monitor moles for any other changes, such as size or shape, and tell your doctor if you notice such changes.

• **Very small outgrowths of skin under your arms or in other places on your body.** Called skin tags, they're caused by skin rubbing against clothing. They often but not always disappear after childbirth. For those that persist and bother you, you can talk to a dermatologist about removal after delivery.

• **Red, itchy palms and soles.** *Palmar erythema* is a hormonal condition. Try added moisturizer made to calm irritated skin. Skin returns to normal after childbirth.

• **Should you develop a rash (red, irritated, or bumpy patches of skin), tell your doctor.** It may simply be the effect of dry skin or stretched skin being rubbed against clothing, for example, or a rash could signal an infection. Best to get it checked to receive the most appropriate care advice.

Mind Update: *WHAT YOU CAN DO NOW TO AVOID POSTPARTUM DEPRESSION*

Postpartum depression (PPD) isn't something any mom-to-be likes to think about—or wants to happen to her. But in fact, it's quite common, affecting up to 10 to 20 percent of new mothers. There are things you can do now, in pregnancy, to help protect yourself against it.

PPD is different from the so-called "baby blues" that affect most new mothers within the first week or so of delivery. That kind of depression seems to go with the territory of shifting post-partum hormone levels, sleep deprivation, recovery, stress, and insecurity, and the anticlimax of pregnancy ending. Where baby blues and weepiness pass within a few days, postpartum depression is more persistent and can be difficult to shake without professional help.

It's not too late to seek help right now if you've been feeling low (or experiencing a return of symptoms from previous depression). Untreated depression now can raise your risk of postpartum depression.

Have you been experiencing . . .

• A constant feeling of disinterest in your baby?

• Extreme irritability or excessive crying?

• A persistent sense of dread or emptiness?

• Inability to concentrate (that goes beyond pregnancy absent-mindedness)?

• Other people in your life (your partner, a friend) commenting on the above? (Others often see signs of depression in us before we recognize it ourselves.)

Tell your provider if you've noticed any of these things. What also helps: A strong support network after your baby arrives. Start working now to line up as large a cross-section of potential helpers as you can—people who can help you with actual baby care or who will simply be available to check in on you and to offer encouragement and support.

Work with your partner to put a postpartum care plan in place—don't assume you can handle it all on your own or that you're a less than "good" mother if you don't. Every new mom needs help! Talk about how you will share childcare and what kind of resources you can tap into to offer added support in the early weeks, such as a meal-delivery service, a cleaning service, or hiring a postpartum doula. If paying for such services yourself is out of the question, consider asking for them as a gift when friends ask, "What do you need for your baby?" Babysitting co-ops, church groups, and the loving hands of friends pitching in together can all be helpful alternatives, so don't hesitate to tap into them. Odds are, excited well-wishers who care about you are standing by just waiting to be asked to help.

DID YOU KNOW that postpartum anxiety is also surprisingly common? It can affect any new mom, and providers increasingly look for both it and postpartum depression, to get affected moms the help they need.

How I'm feeling

Ideas for my postpartum support plan

What I'd like the first week with my baby to look like

Baby brain is real. I should not be permitted to operate heavy equipment, including iPhones.

OLIVIA WILDE

PHOTOS

Week 29

Baby Update

Your baby is now about 15 inches (38.1 cm) long and weighs around 2-3/4 pounds (1.25 kg). The head is getting bigger as the brain grows and develops. The skull remains flexible to enable the head—the largest part of the body—to squeeze through the birth canal, even though the rest of the skeleton begins to harden. It will remain slightly soft in places after birth. A newborn's head has soft spots that you can feel where the skull has not yet fused; they're called *fontanels*.

Your baby's senses are already up and functioning. He can see light and dark, receive sensations from touch, and the taste buds are even well-developed enough that the tastes of sweet and sour are discernible. Perhaps most exciting for you is your baby's hearing ability—your voice, music, and other sounds are already familiar. A very loud noise will cause a startled reflex in the womb.

Body Update: YOUR LEGS

Varicose veins occur when there is a weakness in the veins that carry blood back to your heart from your lower body. Although this condition is often genetic, you can develop them during pregnancy because of hormones, the greater volume of blood being circulated, and the simple fact that there is more weight on your legs.

Varicose veins first look like tiny thin blue, red, or purple lines under your skin. They commonly appear on your legs, ankle, or vulva. You may also feel some pressure or pain in the affected area. They can grow to be thick, raised, or ropey lines and tend to worsen with subsequent pregnancies. In most cases, they're harmless (except to your vanity) and, if you like, may be corrected after you deliver. Call your provider if they begin to cause you severe pain.

These tips can help prevent—or at least reduce—the appearance of varicose veins:

• **Avoid standing or sitting for a long time.**

• **Raise your legs above hip level when you are sitting, when you can, and keep your legs uncrossed.**

• **Place a pillow under your legs when you sleep.**

• **Exercise daily.**

• **Avoid lifting anything heavy.** Review a weight-training regimen with your doctor.

• **Avoid tight pants, socks, and shoes.** Some doctors advise light support/compression hose, putting them on before you get out of bed.

• **Try not to gain more weight than your doctor recommends.**

Mind Update: *THINKING LIKE A MAMA*

A good class on childbirth will help you through delivery—but then what? Use some of your last trimester to pave the way for your transition to motherhood. Knowledge is power, as they say. It's also a great shortcut to confidence.

Some mother prep ideas:

• **Look into breastfeeding support.** It's a natural act, but that doesn't mean it comes naturally to most women. A class can prepare you with techniques, tips, and other resources. Even if you aren't sure whether you will breastfeed, learning what's involved can help you decide. Get the name of a lactation consultant you can call after you deliver.

• **Consider taking a class on baby care.** No amount of reading or even babysitting can prepare you fully for taking care of a little newborn. A class can give you a heads-up on the responsibilities involved and advice on how to handle challenges such as sleep and soothing. Many hospitals offer such classes.

• **Talk with family and friends about their experiences as new parents.** What surprised them most about the transition (in both a good way and a bad way)? What do they wish they had known then? Seek out those who have become new parents recently for the freshest perspectives and tips.

• **Study up on what to expect during your baby's first year, especially the first few months.** You probably won't have time to read in-depth then.

DID YOU KNOW that shortness of breath is a side effect of pregnancy, because your lungs are slightly squished by your expanding uterus?

Thoughts on how we'll handle social media and the baby

Having a baby is like falling in love again, both with your husband and your child.

TINA BROWN

Most surprising symptoms so far

Week 30

Baby Update

We're up to 3 pounds (1.36 kg), 15-1/2 inches (39.4 cm), now. As more space is needed in your nearly stretched-to-the-limit uterus, several things happen. The uterus expands upward, shifting your center of gravity. (This contributes to the swayback posture characteristic of late pregnancy.) The amount of amniotic fluid in the sac also diminishes a bit to make more room for the baby.

The brain—which is one of the body's few organs that won't be fully developed at birth—is changing appearance as it develops. Originally, the surface was fairly smooth, but now distinctive ridges (the *gyri*) and grooves (the *sulci* and deeper fissures) form. These brain folds and wrinkles maximize its surface area within a small space. The brain does most of its "wiring up"—building connections between neurons that affect thinking and learning—in the first year after birth. To support this, from here on, eat lots of DHA, a type of omega-3 fatty acid, to promote vision and thinking skills. Sources: Fatty fish, walnuts, pumpkin seeds.

Body Update: *STEADY ON YOUR FEET*

That awkwardness you may be feeling is rooted in biology: extra weight to manage, loosened ligaments, and a scatterbrained quality that's the result of a preoccupied mind. It's totally natural if you feel a little clumsy.

Here are some tips to avoid bumps, falls, and spills:

• **Take your time getting around.** Don't rush up or down steps, and keep an eye out for obstacles in your way.

• **Keep distractions to a minimum.** Try not to multitask too much—using a phone while driving, for example, is even more risky now than usual.

• **Wear supportive footwear.** Even if high heels didn't bother you earlier, maybe lower their height now. Clogs are a top tripper.

• **Avoid unstable or risky positions.** Standing on one leg, overextending to reach something, or using step stools and ladders should all be avoided.

• **Do some exercise every day.** Even light exercise and stretching can help you gain some balance.

• **If you do fall in late pregnancy, it's a good idea to tell your doctor, even if you feel fine.** She can make a quick check on your baby's well-being.

Mind Update: *A BABY REGISTRY IS NOT A TEST*

Every choice involved in your baby shopping can feel like it has judgments attached. It's easy to get caught up about what this or that brand of diaper or stroller says about you as a parent. Trying to research any one product can send you down a time-sucking rabbit hole. You really don't need to make spreadsheets to analyze the merits of all the options. It's just . . . stuff.

Gentle suggestions:

• **Pick things that look cute or interesting.** Not everything has to be perfect or perfectly enriching.

• **Go with suggestions from family or friends who've been there.** Ask them what they used the most and least.

• **Ask shower guests to give you whatever worked for them.**

• **Remember your baby will keep GROWING.** You'll need clothes in 3-6 month, 6-9 month, and 9-12 month sizes, and children's books you can read now right through preschool.

• **If you're unsure about whether you'll need an item or not, hold off.** There's always overnight delivery if you decide later that something's critical.

DID YOU KNOW that you should discuss a postpartum birth-control plan with your doctor now? You can't know when you'll resume ovulation after giving birth. Don't assume you'll use the same method as you did before, as there may be more suitable options for your life postpartum. And don't assume that breastfeeding will "protect" you from conceiving.

What kind of parents I think we'll be

Thoughts on values

Thoughts on education

Thoughts on discipline

Thoughts on what makes a happy childhood

My body is the site of a miracle now.

KERRY WASHINGTON

Week 31

Baby Update

Your baby is putting on weight more rapidly now—up to about 3-1/2 pounds (1.59 kg), or roughly half of the average birth weight! This gaining trend will last several weeks. Some of this weight is in the form of protective baby fat, which keeps body temperature warm after birth and makes the limbs noticeably plumper. Another consequence of this growth is that space becomes even more scarce, so your baby pulls the limbs closer to the torso in a curl that's known as the "fetal position."

Cool milestone: Around this time, your baby can start using little neck muscles to turn her head from one side to the other.

Body Update: COMFORT CARE FOR LATE-PREGNANCY ICKS

And now a few words about some less-than-jolly side effects of having a baby:

• **Bleeding gums?** Hormonal changes often cause swelling and inflammation, making gums easily irritated, especially when you brush your teeth. But don't put away your toothbrush. Instead, switch to a brush with softer bristles and use a gentler motion. But do continue to brush your gums as well as your teeth, and floss daily. These steps can help you avoid potentially dangerous infections.

• **Sore bottom?** Hemorrhoids, also called piles, occur when veins in your rectum become swollen (making them appear like piles or clusters). The increase in your blood volume during pregnancy makes you more susceptible. You may notice persistent pressure, pain, or itchiness, or sometimes see very slight bleeding. Always inform your doctor of these symptoms to rule out a more serious problem. To prevent and treat hemorrhoids, try relieving pressure from your veins by not standing or sitting in one place for too long. Do Kegels regularly, and include a lot of fluids and high-fiber foods in your diet to help avoid constipation. You may find relief at the site by applying witch hazel (Tucks) pads or taking warm sitz baths. Be careful to keep the area very clean. Never use laxatives or mineral oil to treat hemorrhoids.

• **Bad taste in your mouth?** Because your uterus is squeezing your stomach, its contents may back up into your esophagus, which you notice in your mouth. Smaller servings spread over more mini-meals during the day can do the trick. Drinking water also helps flush your system. It helps to avoid foods liable to irritate your stomach, such as anything fried, creamed, or sauced.

Mind Update: *LOOK GOOD, FEEL GOOD*

Staying true to your style through the homestretch of pregnancy can have a direct effect on how you feel about yourself: positive, peaceful, beautiful.

Some universal pick-me-ups:

• **Your hair.** It's amazing how losing a half inch of hair here and there can make you feel peppier and lighter. Or maybe it's the bliss of sitting back and letting someone else shampoo your scalp and man the blow dryer. If you're leery of a major haircut, still make time for a regular trim to restore a little bounce to your look.

• **Reset your wardrobe.** Yes, you're *almost* to the end, but that doesn't mean your maternity wardrobe should be closed to new things. Buy or borrow a few pick-me-ups; look for stuff that you'll be able to continue wearing postpartum. Many women swear by yoga pants, joggers, or healthcare scrubs (with a tie closure in front) for the final weeks of midsection expansion. Look for roomy tops that can double as nursing shirts, or a voluminous nightgown that will look pretty even after delivery, when you're not filling out so much of the fabric.

• **Jazz up your accessories.** Feel like everyone keeps staring at your midsection when you're trying to carry on a conversation with them? New earrings, necklaces, or a scarf will draw attention from your middle to your face.

• **Try meditation or mindfulness.** If it's not part of your routine now, consider taking 10 or 15 minutes a day to sit still and undisturbed and let your mind wander. Quiet the self-critical "judging" voice in your head, set aside the planning and worrying, and just breathe deeply and empty your thoughts. The peace will show on your face.

• **Go shoe shopping.** You may have a perfectly legitimate excuse, since the same hormone (relaxin) that helps widen your pelvis for delivery also works on the ligaments in your feet. Many women find they need wider shoes or even a half size larger in the last trimester.

DID YOU KNOW that breastfeeding helps your body recover faster from pregnancy? Thank the hormones released, which help shrink the uterus way back.

Three things that are annoying me right now

Three things I'm grateful for now

I just thought, oh, I'm going to hide this forever. But I ended up getting kind of excited to show the bump, as a badge of pride, like, "I'm a woman! Look at me making a human! I am a goddess!"

OLIVIA WILDE

Week 32

Baby Update

Your baby has probably gained a half pound (227 g) in the last week alone, for a total of around 4 pounds (1.81 kg). The skin looks smoother and less red while growing and filling out. Along with storing some fat, he is also building up a good supply of protein, calcium, iron, and other nutrients needed for the final push of growth, and life outside of you. (Coming soon!)

Body Update: *EVERYTHING SWELL?*

There's more than your growing baby to make you feel big. Excess fluid often accumulates in your tissues, so you may notice swelling in your feet or legs and/or your hands. Some swelling, or *edema*, is normal and many pregnant women experience it.

But persistent or marked swelling or the appearance of other symptoms, such as severe headaches, low back pain, vision changes, dizziness, or a surge in your weight gain (over 2 pounds in a week), can signal a more dangerous problem: preeclampsia (formerly called toxemia). Preeclampsia is a syndrome of sudden increased swelling, high blood pressure, and protein in the urine that can be dangerous to mother and fetus. Your doctor or midwife will monitor you for its symptoms, but you should keep watch for them yourself. With timely care, preeclampsia usually can be managed until the baby can be safely delivered. Then the condition disappears.

To help handle ordinary swelling:

• **Choose to sit rather than stand when you can.** When you sit, elevate your feet above hip level whenever possible.

• **Avoid crossing your legs.**

• **Rotate your ankle gently so your foot makes small circles when you're standing or sitting for a while.**

• **Lie down (on your left side) for a while a few times every day.**

• **Drink more fluids, not less, especially water.**

• **Call your doctor if the swelling occurs suddenly, if you experience other symptoms listed above, or if you can't seem to reduce the swelling in 24 hours.** Mention any swelling (even if you're not sure) at your next prenatal checkup.

Mind Update: SHOWER POWER

Some women love being the center of attention at their baby shower. Others dread the very idea of having everybody cluck knowingly and warn them how much their life is about to change. Your feelings about baby showers are no indication of your fitness for motherhood. The fact that friends or family want to throw you a party means they love you and are excited for you.

If you're asked for input, be honest about your preferences. If you don't like silly games, for example, maybe your shower could lean more toward an elegant tea party.

If you're asked what you'd like, do a little research so you can come up with answers that really help you. As you plan a gift registry or list, ask for items you'll need right away, such as a car seat, feeding system, nursing pillow, monitor, baby bathtub, and crib linens. If it's a large shower, include big-ticket choices on your wish list in case two or more friends want to pitch in on a single gift.

At the shower, ask someone to record who gave what, so you don't forget. Try asking guests to share their favorite mothering tips in a notebook. This can be as valuable as anything you might unwrap.

DID YOU KNOW that babies may be programmed to like faces? Not only do they prefer to look at faces when they're born, but also babies in utero seem to prefer light patterns that look like faces as well.

About my baby shower

Date: ....

Who came: ....

....

....

....

....

Gifts: ....

....

....

....

....

Special moments: ....

....

....

....

....

....

All the time we wondered and wondered, who is this person
coming, growing, turning, floating, swimming deep, deep inside?

Crescent Dragonwagon

PHOTOS

Week 33

Baby Update

Your baby is a little over 17 inches (43.2 cm) long and weighs around 4-1/2 pounds (2.04 kg), for another half-pound (227 g) gain in a single week. Her larger size doesn't allow for her previous acrobatic maneuvers—there's simply no room. Instead, movements now tend to consist mostly of nudges, kicks, or jabs.

Although 9 out of 10 babies already settle into a head-down position, the ideal position for birth, smaller babies may continue to rotate for a few weeks more.

Body Update: *NIGHT MOVES*

New sleep difficulties? Simply arranging your body comfortably can be a challenge. And then, no sooner have you drifted off when your bladder—which is being compressed by the expanding uterus—signals the need for you to get up again. Or your baby decides to start practicing for the Rockettes.

• **By day:** Walk or exercise so that when it's time to rest, your body feels ready to drift right to sleep. Fresh air—by going outdoors or opening windows in your home—helps.

• **At bedtime:** Try a small cup of warm milk or chamomile tea to help induce sleep. (Don't worry that it will make you get up to pee; you probably will anyway.) Avoid looking at any screens a few hours before you turn in because the type of light they emit can interfere with sleep.

• **Avoid exercising in the hour or so before bed.** The idea is to wind down.

• **By night:** Continue sleeping on your left side. Make sure your room is not too warm; as you gain weight in the last trimester you are apt to feel warmer than usual. Lower the thermostat or remove heavy blankets.

And speaking of bed, intercourse can't harm your baby, who's well-protected by the uterus. Orgasm won't trigger labor contractions in a healthy woman who's not yet ready to deliver. Getting into a comfortable position is the greater concern (aided by a sense of humor and a willingness to experiment). Remember that intimacy doesn't only mean intercourse. Many couples find oral sex, mutual masturbation, or simple petting and massage to be both erotic and satisfying.

Mind Update: *REWARDS FOR A JOB WELL DONE*

Every week of the last trimester marks an occasion for self-congratulation! Pick a day of the week (Sunday, Friday?) to pat yourself on the back, and treat yourself in some way each week on that day until you deliver.

Some ideas to try:

• **Plan a feel-good outing.** Enjoy a facial or pedicure, get a makeover at a salon or cosmetics counter, or schedule a special prenatal massage.

• **Splurge on a super-comfy throw.** Make it your special nap blanket for the extra sleep you're craving now. You can use it later too, to "sleep when the baby sleeps."

• **Do lunch.** Pick a different friend each week to catch up with over a leisurely meal. Order dessert!

• **Putter.** Spend some time on your favorite hobby or try your hand at something creative like painting pottery at a paint-your-own shop.

• **Take some time off.** Carve out empty space in your calendar to just watch, read, scroll, or listen to some music and let your mind wander.

On my playlist

Movies/TV series watched during pregnancy

What I'm reading

Latest baby name frontrunners (and where they came from)

I feel like a little kid waiting on Christmas for the day I get to meet my baby.

CIARA

Week 34

A baby born prematurely now would have a very good chance of surviving without long-term complications.

Baby Update

Your baby is still shy of an optimal debut: most measure just over 17 inches (43.2 cm) and weigh under 5 pounds (2.27 kg). But survival rates for preemies born at this stage are good, largely because the lungs are now more developed and in rehearsal for breathing outside the womb. Combined with the strengths of modern prenatal care, babies born too soon but who have made it this far can usually beat the odds and grow to live healthy normal lives.

The fingernails and toenails that are growing can be long enough at birth that you'll need to put little mittens and booties on your baby's hands and feet to prevent him from scratching himself.

Body Update: AN EASY LIFT

The closer you get to your due date, the more inclined you may be, on some days, to just drop into the sofa and stay there until somebody wakes you to deliver. You'd be ignoring your body's needs if you didn't just flop down and give yourself a break now and then. At the same time, getting up and moving some every day helps to prepare your body for labor. Exercise also lifts mood and helps you ward off that slow "trapped" feeling.

Aim for easy exercises you can do all day long. Build in more breaks while working to stretch and take long, deep breaths. Sneak in a little walking by dropping off your mail at a mailbox some blocks away, parking farther from the entrance, going up and down the aisles at a big-box store, or window shopping. Stop to rest and hydrate frequently. You may really like swimming now. The buoyancy you feel in the water can be just the relief you're looking for.

Mind Update: YOUR BIRTH PLAN

A birth plan isn't a formal, binding document. It's not even a necessary thing to have. Drafting a simple, easy-to-read document outlining your preferences for labor and delivery does, however, help you think through your options ahead of time and communicate your preferences to those on hand during the birth.

The most effective birth plans are short—about a page—because too much detail is not likely to be remembered or sorted through in the heat of the moment. Besides, you can't control every aspect of your delivery no matter how careful and considered your ideal plan. There are too many variables and unknowns that might come up. That said, it's a great idea to have a general sense of the kind of birth you envision.

A copy of your plan can be placed in your records as a kind of "top-line summary." Be sure to go over your plan with your provider to make sure your desires are clear and your expectations are realistic. Know that hospital policies may affect how your labor is managed, so go over with your doctor areas where your preferences and standard care diverge. Your goal is to be as calm and confident in the delivery room as possible; you don't want to be haggling over practices then.

Some starting questions:

- **What is your attitude toward induction?** Episiotomy? IVs? Electronic fetal monitoring?

- **Who do you want with you when you deliver?** Is there anyone you specifically don't want around?

- **Would you prefer to stay in one place or to move around during labor?** How do you feel about water (shower, bath)?

- **What techniques would you like to try for managing pain?** How do you feel about the various forms of medicated pain relief (epidural, intravenous medication)?

- **What would you like to consume during labor (fluids, small snacks, etc.)?**

- **What position(s) would you like to try during the pushing stage (reclined, sitting, squatting, etc.)?**

- **When would you like the cord cut (immediately or after it stops pulsating) and whom would you like to do it?** Do you want to bank cord blood?

- **How do you prefer to feed your baby?**

- **If the baby is a boy, do you want him circumcised?**

Once you finalize your plan, give a copy to your provider and have a couple of copies ready to take with you to the hospital. Remember this document is not a binding contract. Make sure that your partner and/or labor supporter are on board with your preferences so they can be your ally while you're laboring.

DID YOU KNOW that your uterus expands to 500 times its normal size in pregnancy? (So, that's why you feel so big!)

My vision for the birth

Third trimester thoughts

On the night you were born, the moon smiled with such wonder that the stars peeked in to see you and the night wind whispered, "Life will never be the same."

NANCY TILLMAN, *ON THE NIGHT YOU WERE BORN*

Week 35

Baby Update

Physical development is now almost done, but the "finishing touches"—most important, filling out with protective baby fat—are still underway. This week the average baby is about 18 inches (45.7 cm) long and weighs around 5-1/4 pounds (2.38 kg).

The liver is starting to function, processing waste. Your baby's liver needs to get ready to break down bilirubin, a byproduct of red blood cells. (If it can't do this effectively by the time your baby is born, bilirubin may accumulate in the blood and cause jaundice.) The kidneys are also well developed now. And your baby may be feeling some of your Braxton-Hicks contractions (see page 166), even if you haven't noticed them yet.

Body Update: THE BREAST OF THE STORY

Your bump isn't the only part of your profile that's growing. As your due date nears, you may notice your breasts becoming larger and heavier. Your body is gearing up to nurse your baby. You may even notice a watery clear or yellowish fluid leaking from your nipples. This is colostrum, the "pre-milk" that's especially nutrient- and antibody-rich and will be replaced by regular breast milk (which looks more like cow's milk) a few days after your baby's birth.

To make this new cleavage comfortable, you'll probably need to invest in a new bra or two for more room and adequate support. Check out a good nursing bra, which can serve double duty for now and for later. Look for one that's made of cotton (which is more breathable and doesn't require time-consuming hand-washing), has wide non-elastic straps (for added support without irritation), opens in the front (for nursing—panels that separate are extra convenient), and has expandable cups with no underwire. To keep leaks from showing through your clothing, try disposable or washable breast pads.

Note: The test for Group B Streptococci (Group B strep, or GBS) is usually done via a swab of the vagina and rectum between 35 and 37 weeks. A common bacterium found in one in four moms, GBS can be passed to a baby during birth. It's easily treated by giving the mother IV antibiotics during labor.

Mind Update: WHOM DO YOU WANT AT YOUR DELIVERY?

Mom, Dad, Grandma, Grandpa, midwife, doula, best friend, big sister . . . how many people are too many? You can't really be sure who you'll want in the room until you're in labor. Some women invite a crowd, only to want to be left to primal privacy as labor progresses. Others know they want to leave the sanctity of birth between themselves and their partner alone.

It's your delivery, your choice. You won't be in a state to massage egos, play hostess, arbitrate bickering, or worry about Uncle Bob seeing your stuff. Stick to supportive, low-key people on the invite list. Everybody else can see the baby soon after.

Do consider hiring a doula if your partner feels uneasy about helping you in the delivery room, if there's any chance your chosen labor coach might be traveling or otherwise unavailable when you go into labor, or if you simply think you'd like the extra help. Doula-assisted deliveries have been shown in some research to have shorter labors and fewer complications, possibly because the mothers experience less stress. Note that there are doulas who accompany the mother through labor and delivery, and doulas who provide postpartum care. (Some do both.)

DID YOU KNOW that since the 1970s, some practitioners around the world have used acupuncture to assist with anesthesia in childbirth?

How I expect my life will change

What I'm feeling leery about now

What I'm feeling excited about now

When I was pregnant, I was so huge and people on the bus would get up for me. That made me feel so precious and valued and valuable. I try to treat everyone like they're pregnant.

MARISKA HARGITAY

Week 36

Baby Update

Your baby measures about 18-1/2 inches (47 cm) long and weighs around 6-1/4 pounds (2.83 kg). The layers of creamy vernix and soft lanugo are beginning to come off now as your baby gets ready for life outside the uterus. He swallows these substances with the amniotic fluid, and they become part of the meconium in the bowels. That's the tarry, sticky waste that makes up a newborn's first poops.

It's very likely your baby has settled in the head down, or *cephalic*, position for birth, so brace yourself for some mighty kicks to your ribs. He may also "drop" into position in your pelvis now. If his buttocks or feet sink into the pelvis instead, this is called a breech presentation. Your doctor will have a good idea at this point of how your baby lies.

Body Update: *BRAXTON-HICKS CONTRACTIONS*

You've probably heard of Braxton-Hicks contractions, but you may not know exactly what they are or how to tell you're having them. These involuntary "practice" contractions occur when the muscles of your uterus (which will help push your baby during labor) tighten for 30 seconds to a few minutes and then relax. You may feel or see your abdomen harden, notice a strange squeeze or cramp, or simply sense some pressure. A key way that Braxton-Hicks contractions differ from true contractions is that they don't get longer or closer together over time.

Many women feel these contractions for days to weeks before true labor. In fact, you've probably had them awhile before you ever noticed them. Even though they are painless, they can be slightly uncomfortable. Use them as an opportunity to try out any relaxation techniques you've learned to use during labor. If the contractions become too uncomfortable, try changing position or moving around to reduce your discomfort; they'll almost always stop.

Mind Update: *YOUR BREASTFEEDING PLANS*

Will you, or won't you? How you feed your baby is a personal decision, and it helps to keep an open mind and consider all of the pros and cons as you decide whether to breastfeed, formula feed, or supplement with both.

If you choose to breastfeed, the American Academy of Pediatrics recommends breastfeeding for six months to a year. But you don't have to make a yearlong commitment right off the bat. Take it one day at a time.

Breast milk offers some real benefits. It provides a custom combination of nutrients and a dose of antibodies every day. These protect against infection, illness (now and later in life), and allergies. Breast milk can also be easier to digest than formula, so your baby is less likely to get diarrhea or constipation. The skin-to-skin closeness of breastfeeding provides stimulation and bonding opportunity.

Just like how growing a baby takes a lot of work and energy, so does producing breast milk and feeding around the clock. Give yourself some grace. Having someone who can troubleshoot for you—a friend who has breastfed, a lactation consultant, a nurse—is a big help in the first days.

That being said, for many reasons, not everyone can or wants to breastfeed. Formula feeding is a nutritionally complete, safe, and perfectly valid alternative for you and your baby. It offers convenience, flexibility, and shared opportunities to bond—your partner can take over some feedings, giving them and baby a chance to connect, while you get some time for a much-needed rest.

If you're worried about connecting with your baby during mealtimes, you can still practice skin-to-skin contact while formula feeding. Beyond that, the first months of parenthood offer countless opportunities to strengthen the bond with your baby. Cuddle, sing lullabies, and explore the world together—even if the world is just your backyard. This time goes by fast; the important thing is to enjoy it.

Whatever feeding method you choose, try to remember that it's not all or nothing. You can exclusively breastfeed, exclusively use formula, or use a combination of both. Being a parent is hard work! The world is complicated! As long as you're following medical guidelines, there's no wrong way to feed your baby.

DID YOU KNOW that most hospitals will make sure that you have a properly installed infant car seat before you can leave the hospital with your newborn?

My thoughts about feeding my baby

My support system

There are three reasons for breastfeeding: the milk is always at the right temperature; it comes in attractive containers; and the cat can't get it.

IRENA CHALMERS

Week 37

Hooray! A baby born this week is no longer considered premature or preterm; you've entered the window of a full-term delivery.

Baby Update

Your baby-to-be's hair might be short and fuzzy or rather long—up to 2 inches (5 cm)—and silky soft. Some newborns look bald. This first 'do is not necessarily a look your baby will sport for life, however. Even hair texture and color can change, turning lighter or darker and/or curlier or straighter as it grows.

The irises in the eyes now display color, but it's not necessarily a permanent feature either. They won't lighten or turn bluer, although they often begin as blue and then over the first nine months of life outside the womb, turn to hazel, brown, or a darker blue. Eyes that are light brown at birth may turn dark brown. Average size now: about 19 inches (48.3 cm) long and 6-1/2 pounds (2.9 kg).

Body Update: *TRUE OR FALSE LABOR?*

Wait! Was that IT? Anticipating the contractions that confirm you're in labor when you have never experienced them isn't always easy.

Here are some tips to tell the difference between the start of true labor and a false alarm:

• **Time how long contractions last.** If the length of each one varies a lot and they don't get progressively longer over time, then it's probably false labor. True labor contractions start at around 30 seconds long each and get longer as labor progresses.

• **Time how far apart they occur.** The correct way to measure this is to note the starting time of one contraction and count how many minutes pass until the start of the next. (Don't count the time between the end of one and the start of another.) If the amount of time between contractions is widely inconsistent, then it's probably false labor. True labor contractions follow a pattern, with the time between getting progressively shorter.

• **Locate where you feel the squeeze.** If you feel the contractions in your lower abdomen and/or groin area only, you may be experiencing Braxton-Hicks contractions. Generally, you'll feel true labor contractions higher up, and they'll start to affect your stomach and back as they get stronger and longer.

• **Change position and see if the contractions change.** If they ease up, then it's probably false labor. True labor contractions don't slow down, stop, or feel significantly better with a position change.

• **Might you guess wrong?** Sure. But remember that labor is almost always a lengthy process for a first delivery. It's not likely to "sneak up on you," giving you plenty of time to get to the hospital. In fact, many doctors believe that if you've had a normal pregnancy so far, it's better not to arrive too early at the hospital. Let your body do the work of early labor in the comfort of your own home.

Mind Update: *COMMON LABOR FEARS*

Feeling at least a tiny bit apprehensive about what delivering your baby will be like? It's one of those human experiences that are almost impossible to fully understand and appreciate except by going through them.

Among the common worries of late pregnancy:

• **"What if I can't do it?"** Thoughts along these lines cross everybody's mind: How much will it hurt? Will I say or do something embarrassing? Will I not be able to breathe or push effectively? Fears are normal and real, because you're facing the unknown. You won't be able to plan for or control everything that happens during this natural process. There's no single "right" way to give birth. Prepare yourself as best you can by reading, reviewing your childbirth education notes, or talking to other mothers who had positive birth experiences. And then let it go. Tell yourself that you're going to ride with the experience, trusting in your provider, your body, and your baby to help you along.

• **"Will something go wrong with my baby?"** No matter how many tests or ultrasounds that have indicated all's well, no matter how many times you've heard the baby's strong heartbeat, it can be hard to shake concern for your baby's well-being until the delivery is over. Reassure yourself that the clear majority of newborns are indeed healthy. Even if you're at risk for a particular problem, the odds are in your favor. Confiding your fears to your doctor or genetic counselor can help, especially if they are intense.

• **"What if I'm a terrible mother?!"** Women of all kinds share this rarely spoken fear: those who had good mothers, those who had bad mothers, those who love kids and those who never had any interest in babies or babysat for a single minute of their lives. This type of fear is articulating the opposite: an intense desire to be a good mom. Simply having that intention goes a long way toward making it come true. Remember that babies start out small and grow one day at a time, giving you plenty of opportunity and practice to get up to snuff. You won't need to tackle toilet training, back talk, and how to ride a bicycle right off the bat. And kiss your image of Perfect Motherhood goodbye. There's no such thing. The best part of being a good mother is that you get to define it your own way, not according to anybody else's terms.

DID YOU KNOW that Tuesday is the most popular birth day? Weekends see the fewest deliveries.

My labor hopes

My labor fears

Everything grows rounder and wider and weirder, and I sit here in the middle
of it all and wonder who in the world you will turn out to be.

CARRIE FISHER

Week 38

Baby Update

Although actual stats vary considerably, a standard-sized fetus now measures about 19-1/2 inches (49.6 cm) and weighs around 7 pounds (3.18 kg) at this point. Just how variable are birth weights? A healthy full-term newborn could be a 6-pound (2.72 kg) bantam or a hale 10-pounder (4.54 kg). Both of those would be considered within the normal range.

Most of your baby's lanugo and vernix that once covered the skin have vanished, and she continues to add weight even though she's considered "full term" and, in theory, good to go.

Body Update: SIGNS LABOR IS NEARING

The calendar is telling you the big day is, in theory, any day now. Your body and mind provide you with clues, too. One early sign that labor is drawing near is that your baby "drops" into your pelvis. This is called *lightening*. You may feel pressure or dull pain there or in your upper thighs. You may even look like you're carrying your baby lower than before. Two other external signs are the loss of the mucus plug or your water breaking. The mucus plug seals the opening of your cervix and may become loose as your cervix dilates. When this happens, it looks like a thick bloody discharge or mucus clump. If your water breaks, you may see and feel a gush or a trickle of warm, clear fluid. Although this is a popular sign of impending labor in the movies, it only happens as a first sign of labor about 10 percent of the time. (If it does happen, however, call your provider.) If you've been having Braxton-Hicks contractions, you may notice that you're getting them more frequently. You may also experience soreness in your abdomen or lower back.

You may also feel a surge of energy and an incredible urge to clean up, get organized, and prepare your home for your baby. This instinct is called nesting. Go ahead and heed this primal call, if doing so doesn't stress or overwhelm you. Since you can't know when you'll go into labor, you don't want to squander all your reserves feathering your nest on the night before you'll need that energy to give birth to your little chick.

Call your doctor if:

• **Your water breaks or you are leaking any kind of fluid (even if you think it's maybe just urine).**

• **You notice markedly decreased fetal activity.**

• **Your contractions are 5 to 7 minutes apart (unless your provider advised you of a different timetable).**

• **You just have a strong feeling that you are in labor. Don't feel sheepish about your uncertainty: Trained professionals can quickly determine your labor status and set your mind at ease.**

Mind Update: *ARE YOU PACKED?*

Considering that 80 percent of women have their babies within 2 weeks on one side or the other of their due date, it's smart to get ready for your trip to the hospital now, if you haven't already.

Here are some things you should pack for yourself:

- ☐ Your health insurance card, photo ID, and hospital pre-registration forms
- ☐ A few copies of your birth plan
- ☐ Your childbirth notes (from books or class)
- ☐ Lip balm
- ☐ A pair of warm socks
- ☐ An object you plan to use as your focal point during labor
- ☐ Massage oil and massage tools (such as a tennis ball)
- ☐ Your "goody bag" of relaxation tools for labor
- ☐ A robe and a pair of slippers
- ☐ A nightgown you don't mind getting soiled (and a second one with a front opening if breastfeeding)
- ☐ Toiletries, including extra prescription meds
- ☐ Eyeglasses if you wear them (you probably won't wear contacts all through labor)
- ☐ A hair band or clip
- ☐ Five or more pairs of panties
- ☐ Maxi pads
- ☐ Two bras (nursing bras with front panels if you plan to breastfeed)
- ☐ Your baby book
- ☐ A breastfeeding guide (and/or any notes if you took a class)
- ☐ A comfy outfit for going home (choose one that you wore at about 6-7 months, like leggings and a top that works for breastfeeding)
- ☐ Your phone and other devices and chargers, including an extra-long charger cord to reach from hospital outlet to bed. Portable chargers are also an excellent addition!
- ☐ Earbuds or headphones and/or a portable speaker

- [ ] Favorite pillow from home (optional, but if you do, pick a colorful case to keep it separate from the hospital's so you don't forget it)

- [ ] This *Pregnancy Journal* and pens or pencils!

Here are some things your coach or partner should pack:

- [ ] Snacks and drinks
- [ ] A camera (if you're not just using your phone) and charger
- [ ] A call list in priority order
- [ ] Phone and/or laptop to send updates and/or announcements

- [ ] Playing cards, something to read
- [ ] A great playlist
- [ ] Toiletries

Here are some things to pack for your baby:

- [ ] Some newborn-sized diapers
- [ ] A few newborn-sized outfits; one with legs (to work in car seat; better there than gown-style outfits)
- [ ] A cotton cap

- [ ] Some newborn mittens (to prevent sharp nails from scratching face)
- [ ] A receiving blanket
- [ ] A heavy blanket if it's cold outside
- [ ] An infant car seat

DID YOU KNOW that a newborn's first cries are tearless?

Am I ready?

DELIVERY PACKING LIST

If pregnancy were a book they would
cut the last two chapters.

NORA EPHRON

Week 39

Baby Update

This week a typical fetus is now just shy of 20 inches (50.8 cm) long and 7-1/4 pounds (3.29 kg). In general, boys are born weighing slightly more than girls.

Nobody knows exactly what causes labor to begin, but one theory credits the fetus: It's thought that a hormone deep in the fetal hypothalamus (part of the brain) might set off a chain reaction of events that move from baby to mother, sending her into labor.

Body Update: *LABOR RELAXATION*

A body that's relaxed is better able to work with the force of contractions. The techniques you learned in childbirth education class help you relax in labor. Practice some of these tactics now and they may come to you more naturally in the delivery room.

• **Slow down your breathing, as if you were going to sleep.** Make each inhale deep and full, and on each exhale, drop your shoulders and let the tension roll off.

• **Close your eyes and imagine the work that your body is doing.** During labor, think of each contraction as another big step toward meeting your baby. (You can practice this when you feel Braxton-Hicks contractions.)

• **Ask your coach to give you a massage.** A special massage tool or a regular tennis ball or rolling pin can also help soothe tensed muscles.

• **Concentrate on a focal point.** This could be external, such as an ultrasound image of your baby or a wallpaper pattern, or internal, like imagining holding your baby. In labor, you'll do this for the duration of a contraction. Try practicing while counting to 30, then to 60, then 90. Focus on your chosen image and the numbers you're counting off.

• **Turn on some music.** Whatever helps you relax you or lifts your spirits.

• **Practice mindfulness.** Or play a hypnosis tape if this is a technique that you have used.

• **Visualize a place where you feel comfortable, safe, and happy.** Maybe it's a favorite vacation spot, your childhood home, or your bedroom. If you discuss this with your coach beforehand, he can help describe what you might "see."

• **Take a warm bath or shower** (if your water hasn't yet broken).

Mind Update: A "GOOD" BIRTH

Whether or not you'll have interventions like induction, pain relievers, or a C-section isn't what will make you feel, in the end, like you've had a good delivery. Research based on extensive interviews with mothers shows that instead, these five qualities will be what determines how "good" you feel about how your delivery went:

• **Agency:** The capacity to make your own choices, even if things don't go per your birth plan.

• **Personal security:** How safe you feel during childbirth.

• **Connectedness:** To your providers and birth center staff, to your partner, to other family, to your baby.

• **Respect:** An appreciation that birth is a transformative life event.

• **Knowledge:** Understanding your body and understanding that birth is a process you can't fully control.

These intangible feelings, not specific procedures, are what really color your view of how your baby came into the world.

DID YOU KNOW that U.S. President Woodrow Wilson made Mother's Day official? He signed the order making it a national holiday back in 1914. In the U.K. and Ireland, Mothering Sunday is celebrated on the fourth Sunday of Lent.

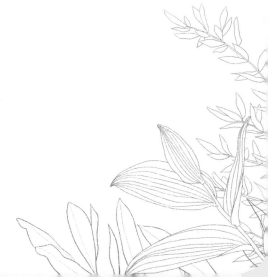

Checking in with my body, mind, and feelings

[Pregnancy] makes me feel like a woman. It makes me feel that all the things about my body are suddenly there for a reason. It makes you feel round and supple, and to have a little life inside you is amazing.

ANGELINA JOLIE

Week 40

Note: Your due date should fall this week.

Baby Update

Average full-term newborn stats:

• **Weight:** 7 pounds, 5 ounces (3.32 kg) (normal range is 6 to 10 pounds, or 2.72 to 4.54 kg)

• **Height:** 20 inches (50.8 cm) (normal range is 18-1/2 to 21-1/2 inches, or 47 to 54.6 cm)

• **Head circumference:** 13.8 inches (35 cm) (normal range is 13 to 14.6 inches, or 33 to 37 cm)

Tall parents tend to have tall children, and short parents tend to have short children. One fun way to guesstimate is the "mid-parent height" formula. Add each parent's height and then divide by 2. Add 2-1/2 inches (6.4 cm) to find the probable adult height of a boy. Or subtract 2-1/2 inches (6.4 cm) to find the probable adult height of a girl.

Body Update: *EARLY LABOR*

Early labor can last a long time, even eight or more hours. During early labor, you will begin to feel contractions at regular intervals, at first about 10 to 20 minutes apart and lasting around 30 seconds. (Some women are not even aware of the first part of early labor, especially if they've given birth before.)

Contractions may cause you some pain or just make you slightly uncomfortable. They will become more intense, but in this phase, you can generally continue to talk and engage in other activities. Gradually contractions move closer together, to about 5 to 7 minutes apart, and longer, to about 40 to 60 seconds long. As you move from early labor to active labor, these contractions tend to demand more concentration from you.

It's generally a great idea, provided your water has not broken, to spend early labor at home. If you get to the hospital too early, you're apt to feel more stressed than relaxed, which works against your body's efforts. Besides, there's not much the medical staff can do for you until your labor is further along.

Some comfort advice for early labor:

• **Time your contractions, both their length and how long between them.** (If it looks like it's taking a while for your contractions to evolve, though, just time them periodically or whenever they seem to be increasing in frequency or intensity.)

• **Pace around your house; go outside.**

• **Put on some music and dance.**

• **Distract yourself with a video, a card game, or some other near effortless activity.**

• **Have a very light, protein-based snack (since you may not want—or be able to have—food later, and you don't know how long your labor will be).** Drink plenty of fluids.

• **Don't overexert.** Save your energy for the later phases of labor.

QUICK REFERENCE:

The Stages of Labor

STAGE ONE: Labor itself.

Early labor (phase 1): Cervix thins (effaces) and dilates to about 3 cm. Most women can still move about and talk easily.

Active labor (phase 2): Cervix dilates to about 7 cm; contractions become longer and require greater concentration (or medication); when most people think of "labor," this is what they mean.

Transition (phase 3): Cervix dilates to its full 10 cm; contractions are long with several "peaks" and run together; this stage is intense but relatively brief.

STAGE TWO: Delivery of the baby (a.k.a. "pushing").

STAGE THREE: Delivery of the placenta.

Mind Update: PREOCCUPIED

When you're this great with child, it's hard to think about much else besides your pregnancy: When will your labor begin? How will you know? What will you do? What will it be like? What will your baby be like? What will being a mother be like?

These thoughts can manifest in many ways. You may find that your mood swings are more rapid and intense. You may feel anxious, fretful, or just plain tired. Other times you may feel calm, excited, and ready. Your relationship may feel closer or more strained—neither of you can exactly understand the unique stresses of the other, and at the same time you're each preoccupied by those stresses. Add to all this the fact that well-wishers seem to be calling and asking every hour how it's going and whether anything's "happening" yet.

Look for ways to take your mind off waiting. Go see a matinee or binge-watch a hit show. Listen to podcast after podcast. Dig out your favorite novel and reread it. Do some yoga or meditation, since the whole point of these activities is to let go of all the thoughts crowding your brain. Have lunch with a friend who promises not to say one word about the baby for one full hour. It's not that you can forget you're pregnant, but by purposefully turning your attention elsewhere for a while, you can find some much-needed relaxation.

DID YOU KNOW that it's not true that only firstborns are usually late? More than half of all babies are born after their projected due dates; 35 percent arrive before the due date and 5 percent hit D-day perfectly.

HEADLINES:
WHAT'S HAPPENING
IN THE WORLD RIGHT NOW

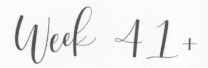

Week 41+

Body Update: HANGING IN THERE

As you move past your due date, your doctor will monitor your baby carefully to make sure all's well. These tests can show whether the baby is still moving well in the uterus and whether there is sufficient amniotic fluid. Possible tools include the non-stress test, contraction stress test, biophysical profile, and ultrasound. Your own vital signs will also be watched.

Whether you're induced is a question that's based on your and your baby's perceived health, the perceived accuracy of your LMP and due dates, and whether there are signs of impending labor. It's not a decision to be made lightly, so be sure that you understand the reasons why an induction is recommended or not.

A "late" baby is still right on time for him or her!

Make use of your "found" time:

• Soothe an aching back with a massage or a hot water bottle.

• Return any baby shower items you don't want or need for store credit.

• Hire a childproofing service to get your home ready, or follow a checklist for how to do it.

• Do pelvic tilts to alleviate back pain or pressure in your lower abdomen and groin area.

• Take warm showers or baths for an all-over refresher—and there's no rule you should only do so once a day.

• Stock the pantry with nonperishables like tuna, beans, other canned goods, bath tissue, detergent, paper towels.

• Order a crib nightlight if you haven't already received one—it's genius.

• Get a pedicure. Soon, you'll be able to see those toes again!

• Keep your car fueled up.

Mind Update: "HAVE YOU TRIED . . . ?"

You may be short on labor pains, but there's one thing bound to be in plentiful supply as your due date comes and goes: tips and tricks from friends, loved ones, and perfect strangers for how to induce labor.

Most of these, alas, are old wives' tales. They're unproven, unfounded, and unlikely to work. If they're harmless, though, hearing them (and even trying them, if you're in the mood) can provide entertainment to pass these last days.

So, have you tried . . .

Eating spicy food? Walking with one foot on a curb and one foot in the street? Eating pizza, meat loaf, Chinese food, or pickles? A teaspoon of castor oil? Drinking Grandma's favorite tea brew? Having sex? (There's a smidgen of truth in that last one, since the oxytocin released during arousal and orgasm can trigger contractions in a woman who's ready to deliver—but there's no surefire cause-and-effect relationship between sex and labor.)

DID YOU KNOW that technically a baby is not "overdue" until two weeks after your due date? Most babies today, however, are delivered before they are officially "postdates."

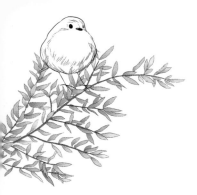

YOUR FAMILY TREE

You!

_____
YOUR NAME!
_____
BIRTH DATE & PLACE

your parents

_____
ME, YOUR MOTHER!
_____
BIRTH DATE & PLACE

_____
NAME
_____
BIRTH DATE & PLACE

your grandparents

_____
NAME
_____
BIRTH DATE & PLACE

_____
NAME
_____
BIRTH DATE & PLACE

_____
NAME
_____
BIRTH DATE & PLACE

_____
NAME
_____
BIRTH DATE & PLACE

your great-grandparents

_____
NAME
_____
BIRTH DATE & PLACE

_____
NAME
_____
BIRTH DATE & PLACE

_____
NAME
_____
BIRTH DATE & PLACE

_____
NAME
_____
BIRTH DATE & PLACE

_____
NAME
_____
BIRTH DATE & PLACE

_____
NAME
_____
BIRTH DATE & PLACE

_____
NAME
_____
BIRTH DATE & PLACE

_____
NAME
_____
BIRTH DATE & PLACE

My feelings

It's been the most amazing experience I could ever possibly imagine.
How any woman does what they do is beyond comprehension.

PRINCE HARRY, DUKE OF SUSSEX

Your Labor and Delivery

Bring this journal to the hospital with you so that you can record what happened while the details are still very fresh in your mind. Your labor and delivery experience is also your child's birth story. If you don't have time to record a full description of the day's (and/or night's) events, take a few minutes to at least jot down some notes about the highlights. They will jog your memory so that you can go back and explore the big event in more depth and detail later, if you wish.

Research shows that women who spend time processing and sharing their labor stories—no matter how difficult or easy the experience—tend to have happier memories and feel more satisfied and proud of the event. Seek out people with whom you can share your story. Write and think about it. Turn it over in your head. Yes, it's that big a deal!

Your body does something truly amazing and wonderful in creating a new life. Celebrate that singular fact! Feel proud of yourself and your accomplishment, whether or not everything unfolded the way you hoped or wished. Less than half the population ever does what you did!

How and when I first thought I might be in labor

How I got to the hospital

What happened once I arrived

Progress of labor (high points, results of labor checks, length of labor stages)

What helped most

What didn't help or appeal to me

What was hardest

What was best

How it was what I expected

How it was not what I expected

How long labor lasted overall

Meeting my baby

Who was there

How I feel now

Welcome to the world

BABY BASICS

Full name

Date of birth

Time of birth

Length

Weight

Head circumference

Attendants

Hair color

Eye color

Distinctive marks

Baby looks like

How we told the world

Baby's first visitors

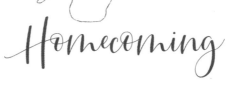

Homecoming

Day we came home

Where baby slept

Who visited at home

What's happening in the world right now

What names will the grandparents go by?

I remember leaving the hospital thinking,
"Wait, are they going to let me just walk off with him?"

ANNE TYLER

PHOTOS

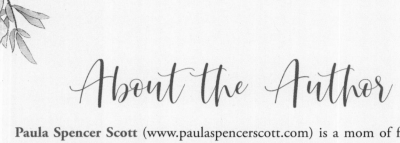

About the Author

Paula Spencer Scott (www.paulaspencerscott.com) is a mom of four and stepmom of two, and the author of a dozen books about women's health, family, pregnancy, and parenting, including *Like Mother, Like Daughter* and *Mother and Son: Our Back-and-Forth Journal* (both from Peter Pauper Press). She also co-authored Dr. Harvey Karp's *The Happiest Toddler on the Block*. Scott lives in Fort Collins, Colorado.

Index

Notes

Notes

Notes

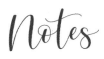

Notes

Notes

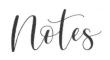

Notes

PHOTOS • MEMORIES • MEMORABILIA